HEALING REVOLUTION

A passionate believer in Ayurveda and a regular practitioner of yoga, **Ram K. Sharma** is Managing Director of Baidyanath, an Ayurvedic and herbal medicine manufacturing company going back over 100 years. He also serves as a Board Member of 10 companies and is a former Board Member of South Asia Young Presidents' Organization (YPO).

After schooling from Delhi's Modern School, Barakhamba Road, he did B.Com (Honours) from the prestigious Shri Ram College of Commerce, Delhi University. He also holds an MBA degree from Fairleigh Dickinson University, New Jersey, USA.

A keen sportsman, Ram Sharma captained his school and college field hockey teams. He is a regular practitioner of Kriya Yoga, a form of meditation revived by Shri Paramahansa Yogananda.

He lives in Kolkata with his wife Rashmi and has three children.

HEALING REVOLUTION

Defeat 100 Ailments with Ayurveda, Yoga and Lifestyle

Ram K. Sharma

RUPA

Published by
Rupa Publications India Pvt. Ltd 2025
161-B/4, Gulmohar House,
Yusuf Sarai Community Centre,
New Delhi 110049

Sales centres:
Bengaluru Chennai
Hyderabad Kolkata Mumbai

Copyright © Ram K. Sharma 2025

The views and opinions expressed in this book are the author's own and the facts are as reported by him; these have been verified to the extent possible, and the publishers are not in any way liable for the same.

While every effort has been made to verify the authenticity of the information contained in this book, it is not intended as a substitute for medical consultation with a physician. The publisher and the author are in no way liable for the use of the information contained in this book.

All rights reserved.
No part of this publication may be reproduced, transmitted, or stored in a retrieval system, in any form or by any means, electronic, mechanical, photocopying, recording or otherwise, without the prior permission of the publisher.

P-ISBN: 978-93-6156-663-9
E-ISBN: 978-93-6156-134-4

Second impression 2025

10 9 8 7 6 5 4 3 2

The moral right of the author has been asserted.
Printed in India
This book is sold subject to the condition that it shall not, by way of trade or otherwise, be lent, resold, hired out, or otherwise circulated, without the publisher's prior consent, in any form of binding or cover other than that in which it is published.

*Dedicated to my loving family:
my wife Rashmi, my children, their spouses, and
my grandchildren.*

Contents

Preface	*xi*
Introduction	*xiii*

1. Anaemia — 1
2. Acne — 3
3. Anorexia (Loss of Appetite) — 5
4. Anxiety — 7
5. Arthritis — 10
6. Bronchitis and Asthma — 13
7. Backache — 15
8. Boils — 18
9. Bleeding Gums — 21
10. Breast Milk Insufficiency — 25
11. Constipation — 28
12. Common Cough — 31
13. Colitis: Inflammation of the Colon — 34
14. Cystitis (Inflammation of the Urinary Bladder) — 37
15. Cataract — 39
16. Cervical Spondylosis — 41
17. Chickenpox (*Laghu Masurika*) — 44
18. Cramps — 47
19. Conjunctivitis — 50
20. Diabetes Mellitus — 52
21. Dyspepsia — 55
22. Dysentery — 57
23. Dandruff (Scaliness of the Scalp) — 60
24. Depression — 63
25. Diarrhoea — 65

26. Epilepsy	67
27. Eczemas	70
28. Enlarged Prostate	73
29. Flatulence	76
30. Fatigue	78
31. Fever	81
32. Female Sterility	83
33. Gout	86
34. Gastritis	88
35. Gallstones	91
36. Goitre	95
37. Greying of Hair	97
38. General Debility	99
39. Gonorrhoea	102
40. Hypercholesterolemia (High Cholesterol)	104
41. Hyperacidity	106
42. High Blood Pressure (Hypertension)	108
43. Hair Loss	110
44. Hiccups	113
45. Haemoptysis	115
46. Heart Disease	117
47. Indigestion	120
48. Insomnia	122
49. Immunity Disorders	124
50. Influenza	126
51. Intestinal Worms	128
52. Irregular Menstrual Periods	130
53. Jaundice and Hepatitis	133
54. Joint and Muscle Pain	135
55. Kidney Stones	138
56. Leucorrhoea	141
57. Leukoderma	143
58. Low Blood Pressure	146
59. Liver Disorder	148

60. Male Sterility — 150
61. Miscarriage and Abortion — 152
62. Menorrhagia — 154
63. Myopia — 156
64. Memory Loss — 158
65. Migraine (Severe Headache with Nausea) — 161
66. Measles — 164
67. Obesity — 166
68. Oedema — 168
69. Perimenopause — 170
70. Piles — 175
71. Premenstrual Syndrome (PMS) — 177
72. Pyorrhoea — 179
73. Psoriasis (Scaly Disorder of the Skin) — 182
74. Peptic Ulcer (Stomach Ulcer) — 184
75. Prostate Disorder — 187
76. Palpitations — 190
77. Painful Menstruation — 192
78. Premature Ejaculation — 195
79. Premature Baldness — 197
80. Rheumatism — 199
81. Ringworm — 201
82. Sinusitis — 203
83. Skin Care — 205
84. Sore Throat — 207
85. Sexual Impotence — 209
86. Stomach Ulcer — 211
87. Skin Allergy — 213
88. Sciatica — 216
89. Syphilis — 218
90. Sleeplessness — 220
91. Stress — 222
92. Tonsillitis (Inflammation of the Tonsils) — 226
93. Toothache — 228

94.	Underweight (Less than Normal Weight)	230
95.	Urinary Tract Diseases	234
96.	Urticaria	238
97.	Vertigo	241
98.	Women and Obesity	243
99.	Warts (Superficial Growths on the Skin)	246
100.	Whooping Cough	248

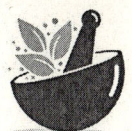

Preface

In today's fast-paced world, where stress, unhealthy diets, and sedentary habits have become the norm, maintaining good health can seem like a challenge. While modern medicine offers solutions for treating diseases, it often overlooks the importance of prevention and overall wellbeing. Ayurveda, yoga and a balanced lifestyle provide a holistic approach to staying healthy and disease-free—an approach that I have personally followed for years with great success.

This book is born out of my own experience. I have used the ancient sciences to maintain my health, prevent illness and live with vitality. Ayurveda teaches us how to align with nature's rhythms, to eat according to our unique constitution, and to use herbs and daily routines to support our wellbeing. Yoga strengthens the body, calms the mind and enhances overall energy. A mindful lifestyle ties everything together, helping us create habits that nourish and sustain us in the long run.

Through this book, I want to share practical, easy-to-follow guidance on how you too can integrate these time-tested practices into your daily life. Whether you are new to Ayurveda and yoga or looking to deepen your knowledge, this book will provide insights, tools and techniques to help you take charge of your health naturally.

True wellness is not just the absence of disease—it is a state of balance, energy and joy. I invite you to join me on this journey and discover how Ayurveda, yoga and conscious living can transform your health and life.

Swami Vivekananda had emphasized the importance of good health thus:

'First of all, our young men must be strong. Religion will come afterward. Be strong, my young friends; that is my advice to you. You will be nearer to Heaven through football than through the study of the Gita. These are bold words; but I have to say them, for I love you. I know where the shoe pinches. I have gained a little experience. You will understand the Gita better with your biceps, your muscles, a little stronger. You will understand the mighty genius and the mighty strength of Krishna better with a little strong blood in you. You will understand the Upanishads better and the glory of the Atman when your body stands firm upon your feet, and you feel yourselves as men. Thus we have to apply these to our needs.'

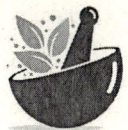

Introduction

Ayurveda and yoga are deeply connected practices that originate from Indian Vedic science. The strength of Ayurveda and yoga lies in the way the disease is treated. Patients are treated based on their Ayurvedic body (*dosha*) and not just the ailment. As each body is different, it should be treated likewise with a combination of herbs, medicines, yoga, diet control and lifestyle changes.

Healing is a deeply personal journey that requires not only addressing symptoms, but also understanding the root causes of imbalance in the mind, body and spirit. In this fast-paced modern world, we often lose touch with our naturally healthy bodies, leaving us vulnerable to a wide range of physical and emotional ailments. The ancient sciences of Ayurveda, yoga and mindfulness offer profound solutions—tailored, holistic and rooted in nature.

This book is a guide to healing 100 common ailments using the time-tested principles of Ayurveda, the transformative power of yoga, and practical lifestyle changes. From digestive issues and stress to skin disorders and chronic fatigue, this book offers natural remedies and tools to help you restore balance and vitality. Each ailment is addressed with specific dietary advice, herbal remedies, yoga practices and daily routines that not only alleviate symptoms but also promote long-term well-being.

The power of this approach lies in its simplicity and effectiveness.

Ayurveda teaches us that every individual is unique and that healing requires a personalized approach. Yoga complements this wisdom by connecting the body, mind and breath, creating a space for transformation from within. Together, these practices help to reawaken the body's innate intelligence and self-healing ability.

According to Ayurvedic principles, any imbalance in the three *doshas* leads to ailments—at least eighty types in case of imbalanced *vata*, forty for an imbalanced *pitta*, and another twenty in case of *kapha* being out of balance.

The following chart will give you some indications of the problems that one is likely to face in each case:

Vata Ailments	**Pitta Ailments**	**Kapha Ailments**
Pain in the feet	Burning	Anorexia nervosa
Stiffness of the ankle	Acid excretion	Drowsiness
Cramps in the calf	Burning sensation in the chest	Lack of sleep
Sciatica	Burning sensation in the body	Heaviness of the body
Paraplegia	Foul odour of the body	Excess mucus production
Rectal prolapse	Urticaria	Indigestion
Stiffness of the back	Genital herpes	Mucus in the throat
Chest pain	Jaundice	Atherosclerosis or narrowing of the arteries
Gripping abnormal pain	Excessive thirst	Goitre
Stiff neck	Pharyngitis	Obesity
Toothache	Conjunctivitis	
Cataract	Inflammation of the penis	
Headache	Skin warts	
Dandruff		
Facial paralysis		
Monoplegia		

Violent muscular convulsions	
Giddiness	
Hiccups	
Weakness	
Mental instability	

This book is not just a collection of remedies; it is an invitation to embark on a deeper journey of self-awareness and empowerment. By integrating these ancient practices into your daily life, you can address not only the ailments themselves but also the lifestyle patterns that may contribute to them.

Whether you are new to Ayurveda and yoga, or already familiar with their benefits, this book offers practical, actionable steps to enable you to take charge of your health. Let it be your companion and guide, helping you rediscover the harmony and vitality that are your birthright.

With warmth and healing
—Ram K. Sharma

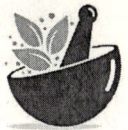

1
Anaemia

Termed *pandu* in Ayurveda, anaemia is a very common ailment, where the haemoglobin and red blood cells (RBCs) count falls from its normal level of 15 g of haemoglobin per 100 ml of blood and approximately 5 million RBCs per cubic millimetre of blood.

Symptoms

- Weakness, dizziness and quick exhaustion
- Haggard look lined with premature wrinkles
- Eyes stripped off their shine, mirroring fatigue
- Failing memory
- Shortness of breath and heart palpitations
- Occasional headaches
- Slow healing of wounds
- Pale-looking skin and mucous membranes

Root Causes

- Loss of blood from the body because of haemorrhaging via injury, bleeding piles, bleeding from the nose, mouth, lungs, anus, genital tracts, or excessive menstruation in case of women
- Inadequate supply of blood-forming ingredients in food
- Destruction of RBCs inside the body
- Poor blood formation because of malfunctioning liver or bone marrow issues

- Lack of hydrochloric acid in the stomach needed for the digestion of iron and proteins
- Presence of hookworms, pinworms, roundworms and tapeworms that feed on the supply of blood and vitamins

Healing Options

Home Remedies	• Punarnava (*Boerhavia diffusa*) • Ghritkumari (Aloe vera)
Ayurvedic Supplements	• Dhatri lauh • Navayas lauh • Lohasava • Lauh Bhasma
Diet	Go for a well-balanced diet rich in iron. Eat sesame seeds, almonds, dairy products, animal protein, vegetables like beetroots, lettuce and spinach, soya beans, radish, carrots, tomatoes, and fresh fruits like bananas, blackberries, strawberries, apples, amla and plums.
Lifestyle	Enjoy sunbathing as the sunlight stimulates the production of red blood cells.
Yoga	• Sarvangasan (Shoulder stand) • Paschimottanasan (Posterior stretch) • Shavasan (Corpse pose) • Padahastasan • Vajrasan • Viparita Karani with wall support

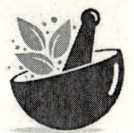

2
Acne

Acne is an inflammatory condition of the sebaceous glands and hair follicles which primarily affects teenagers.

Symptoms

Blackheads, pimples, small superficial sebaceous cysts, and scars on the forehead, temples, cheeks, chin, chest, back and, in rare cases, the whole body

Root Causes

- Eating at irregular hours, excessive consumption of starchy, sugary, fried and fatty food
- Toxins (*ama*) formed due to improper movement of the bowels, finding their way into the bloodstream
- Unhygienic living habits
- Excessive intake of tea, coffee, alcohol or tobacco

Healing Options

Home Remedies	• Cinnamon, sandalwood and turmeric for local application • Neem (*Azadirachta indica*) • Giloy (*Tinospora cordifolia*)

| Ayurvedic Supplements | • Neem Guard Capsules
• Surakta Syrup
• Surakta Tablets
• Mahamanjishthadyarishta
• Haridra Khand |
|---|---|
| Diet | • Avoid eating excess meat, sugar, tea or coffee, condiments, pickles, soft drinks, candies, ice cream, refined and processed food.
• Have lemon juice, coriander soup, mint juice and water.
• Opt for a fat-free diet with plenty of green salads and fruits. |
| Lifestyle | • Apply crushed orange peel, fenugreek paste or a mixed paste of sandalwood and turmeric to the affected area.
• Wash your face with lukewarm water and neem-based soap thrice a day. |
| Yoga | • Simhasan (Lion pose)
• Kapalabhati
• Gomukhasan
• Halasan |

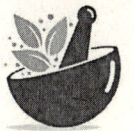

3

Anorexia (Loss of Appetite)

Anorexia is an eating disorder that causes weight loss. It is a symptom of poor digestion and a common result of failure of stomach activity and secretion of gastric juices due to low vitality, which in turn can be due to various causes.

A person suffering from this disease may refuse to eat. They might also suffer from insomnia.

Symptoms

- Refusing to eat
- Dehydration, fainting, fatigue, low blood pressure
- Fear of gaining weight

Root Causes

People suffering from anorexia habitually take a poor diet and rarely exercise. It can also be caused by mental or domestic stress or emotional disturbances. Difficult working conditions and nervous disorders may also cause anorexia.

Healing Options

Home Remedies	• Lime • Ginger • Garlic • Orange • Apple
Ayurvedic Supplements	• Agnitundi Bati • Kshudhakari Bati • Amlaki Rasayan
Diet	• The only effective treatment for anorexia is cleansing the digestive tract and adopting a sensible diet thereafter, along with a lifestyle change. • Fruits like apples, pears, grapes, oranges, pineapples and peaches are helpful. • The person should adopt a restricted diet of easily digestible food, consisting of lightly cooked vegetables, juicy fruits and buttermilk.
Lifestyle	During the first three to five days of the juice fast, the bowels should be cleansed with a warm water enema every day. The poisonous matter will be eliminated by this self-cleansing process.
Yoga	• Padmasan (Lotus pose) • Pranayam (Breathing exercises) • Vajrasan • Ardha Kurmasan • Dhanurasan

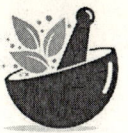

4

Anxiety

Anxiety is an emotional state of uneasiness and distress, or a feeling of impending doom, although there is no obvious threat. It is characterized by apprehension and worry. Experiencing some anxiety is normal, but it becomes a problem when it interferes with everyday activities. According to Ayurveda, anxiety is a classic sign of imbalance in the body. Prolonged anxiety and stress affect the nervous system and can cause further complications if ignored.

Ayurveda, the 'science of life', provides a clear, concise and cohesive regimen to help people cure anxiety naturally. Yet, it is much more than just an effective holistic treatment. It provides a complete system of preventive medicine and health care that has proven its effectiveness over thousands of years in India.

Root Causes

- Negative thinking
- General weakness
- Prolonged malnutrition
- Family or personal issues
- Fears
- Stress
- Menstrual disorders in women

Symptoms

- Headache
- Inability to relax
- Sleeplessness
- Heart palpitations
- Tightness in the chest
- Belching, nausea and occasional diarrhoea
- Emotional instability
- Tendency to be irritable without an obvious cause
- Tendency to cry without an obvious reason

Healing Options

Home Remedies	**Managing anxiety with yoga** Before starting yoga practice to control anxiety, stay in the corpse pose for ten minutes. Use this time to mentally detach from past experiences and the anticipated events (real or imaginary) of the future. **Managing anxiety with breathing exercises** Lie on your back in a comfortable place. Breathe in slowly through your nose. Use your diaphragm to fill air in your lungs and at the same time, allow your belly to expand. After your belly is fully stretched, continue to inhale as deeply as possible. Reverse the process while breathing out. Contract your belly while exhaling slowly and completely. Repeat this exercise several times.
Ayurvedic Supplements	- Anti-stress massage oil - Stress Guard - Shankhpushpi Syrup - Ashwagandha capsules

Lifestyle	Don't procrastinate, hide, or run away. Believe that you have the power to overcome your anxiety. It may not immediately feel good to face the fear directly, but if this strategy is applied consistently, it always works. Often, anxiety is rooted in exaggeration of one's worst fears and negative thoughts. If you are the kind of person who embraces 'worst-case scenarios' regularly, you may need a cognitive tune-up. Strategies such as thought-stopping might be helpful. Whenever a negative or an anxious thought occurs, such as 'I'm going to make a fool of myself' or 'I don't measure up', tell yourself to STOP! Stopping these thoughts is essential for interrupting the cycle of anxiety.
Yoga	• Tadasan • Vrikshasan • Tuladandasan

5
Arthritis

Arthritis broadly refers to the conditions that affect the joints and the surrounding connective tissues. Swelling and inflammation of one or more of the joints results in stiffness and pain, which in turn makes movement painful and difficult.

According to Ayurveda, arthritis, or *amavata*, is triggered by the imbalance or vitiation of vata along with the accumulation of toxins in the joints. This accumulation is the result of poor digestion and metabolism. As such, the treatment for amavata generally involves balancing the vata, while eliminating ama from the body.

Arthritis is differentiated into two main types—osteoarthritis and rheumatoid arthritis.

Osteoarthritis is the more common type and is caused by the progressive wearing away of the cartilage that caps the bones in the joints.

Rheumatoid arthritis, on the other hand, is an autoimmune disease in which the body's own immune system attacks the joints, causing inflammation.

Symptoms

- Joint pain
- Stiffness and tenderness of the joints
- Limited range of motion
- Weakness
- Red skin over the affected area

Healing Options

Home Remedies	• **Garlic:** The most important home remedy for arthritis is garlic. Oil prepared from garlic and rubbed on the affected area will give great relief. The patient may thereafter take a warm-water bath. This treatment should be continued for at least 15 days. • **Shallaki:** This herb strengthens the joints from within and alleviates pain. It also helps in diminishing the swelling and increases mobility. • **Ginger:** It is known for its exceptional antiseptic and anti-inflammatory properties that help reduce joint pain and swelling. It is also known to increase blood circulation, which can help cut down pain in the affected areas. • **Turmeric:** This is another effective and natural remedy that is used to treat chronic arthritis. The use of turmeric can considerably lessen joint pain in people with arthritis. Turmeric contains curcumin, which has superior anti-inflammatory properties.
Ayurvedic Supplements	• Arthplus • Arthoil • Rhumatho • Rhumartho Gold • Yograj Guggul • Lakshadi Guggul **Massage Oils** • Rhuma Oil for light massage • Mahanarayan Oil for regular massage

Diet	• The diet of those suffering from arthritis should consist of a salad of raw vegetables such as tomato, carrot, cabbage, cucumber, radish, lettuce and at least two steamed or lightly cooked vegetables such as cauliflower, cabbage, spinach, carrot, and plenty of fruits except bananas. • The patients should avoid fatty, spicy and fried food, curd, sweetmeats and sugar, condiments, tea and coffee. • Processed food has few nutrients and should be eliminated from the diet.
Lifestyle	• Smoking or tobacco in any form should be given up completely. Hot fomentation, alternate sponging, or application of heat to the affected area will also provide immediate relief.
Yoga	• Bhujangasan • Shalabhasan • Halasan • Paschimottasan

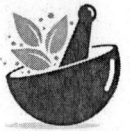

6

Bronchitis and Asthma

In Ayurveda, bronchial asthma is an allergic condition resulting from the reaction of the body to one or more allergens and is one of the most fatal respiratory diseases. It is called *tamaka shwasa* and its seat of manifestation is the lungs.

Symptoms

During a bronchial asthma attack, one has to gasp for air—breathing out is more difficult than breathing in as the air cannot be properly driven out of the lungs before the next breath. Chronic patients encounter frequent attacks, especially in the night or early morning, often preceded by nasal congestion and sneezing.

Root Causes

Bronchial asthma can be caused by allergy-inducing factors such as weather, dust, food, drugs, perfumes, pollution, or psychological factors like deep-seated emotional insecurity, an intense need for parental love, or hereditary or genetic factors.

Healing Options

Home Remedies	• Tulsi (*Ocimum sanctum*) • Vasaka (*Adhatoda vasica*)
Ayurvedic Supplements	• Vasavaleh • Kanakasava • Talisadi Churna • Kantakaryavaleha • Swasa Kalpa
Diet	• Limit intake of carbohydrates, fats and proteins. • Eat a liberal amount of alkaline food like fresh fruits, green vegetables, sprouted seeds and grains. • Avoid food that tends to produce phlegm, such as rice, sugar, lentils and curd. • Avoid difficult-to-digest food like strong tea, coffee, alcoholic beverages, condiments, pickles, sauces and all refined and processed food.
Lifestyle	• Avoid excess humidity. • Avoid exposure to dust, fumes and pollen. • Check allergens.
Yoga	• Ardha Kati Chakrasan • Dhanurasan • Ustrasan • Ardha Kurmasan

7
Backache

Backache is one of the most common afflictions. It is the most agonizing and incapacitating physical disorder and owes its origin to multiple physical factors.

It is merely a symptom and not a disease, the cause of which lies elsewhere in the body. The spine of the human body is comprised of cervical vertebrae, thoracic or dorsal vertebrae, lumbar vertebrae, sacrum and coccyx or tailbone. During backache, only the lumbar portion is affected, although the pain may also radiate to the sacrum and coccyx.

Symptoms

- Constant pain, at times unbearable and severe
- Difficulty bending forwards and sideways
- Aggravation of pain with minimal movement or jerks
- Soreness and sensitivity to even the slightest touch
- Relief with gentle massage
- Incapacitation
- Tightness of back muscles

Root Causes

- Sitting in a particular position at a stretch, but more often when one is obliged to perform a job where bending of the back is necessary
- Spinal arthritis, rheumatoid or ankylosing spondylitis
- Curvature of the spine
- Tumours in the spine
- Chronic infection
- Injury to the spine or abnormal stress caused by lifting heavy objects
- Poor blood circulation
- Psychological upsets

Healing Options

Home Remedies	- Garlic (*lehsun*) - Lemon - Guggul - Ginger
Ayurvedic Supplements	- Arth Plus - Arth Oil - Yograj Guggulu - Rumartho Gold Plus - Rhuma Oil
Diet	- The diet of those suffering from backache should consist of a salad of raw vegetables like tomatoes, carrots, cabbages, cucumbers, radish, lettuce and at least two steamed or lightly cooked vegetables like cauliflowers, cabbages, spinach, carrots, and plenty of fruits except bananas. - The patient should avoid fatty, spicy or fried food, curd, sweetmeats, sugar, condiments, tea and coffee.

	• Food processed for preservation has few nutrients and should be eliminated from the diet.
Lifestyle	• Smoking or taking tobacco in any form should be given up completely.
	• Hot fomentation, alternate sponging, or application of heat to the back provides immediate relief.
Yoga	• Bhujangasan
	• Shalabhasan
	• Halasan
	• Savasan
	• Pawanmuktasan
	• Eka Pada Salavasan

8
Boils

Boils are localized, tender, inflamed and pus-filled lumps in the skin surrounded by large red areas. They are infections of the hair follicles of the skin. Boils are quite painful, particularly in areas where the skin is closely attached to the underlying tissues, such as the nose, ears or fingers. They usually occur in teenagers and young adults. The common sites for boils are the face, neck and thighs.

Symptoms

At first, a painful red nodule appears on the skin. This grows bigger and then ruptures where the pus collects. The painful red nodular area experiences a great deal of irritation and itching. There may be a single boil, or several boils in the same area or in different areas at the same time. The swelling may not be limited to one hair follicle, but extend to several follicles. When boils ripen, they release pus. Fever may sometimes accompany the boils.

Root Causes

Boils may be caused by staphylococcus bacteria entering the sweat glands or hair follicles. The main cause of boils is thus bacteria. However, several factors predispose the growth of bacteria in hair follicles. Of these, the chief one is a toxic condition in the bloodstream, which is due to a poor diet and a frenetic pace of living. Boils generally appear when a person is in a run-down and devitalized condition.

Healing Options

Home Remedies	• Garlic • Onion • Betel leaves • Cumin seeds • Neem leaves • Turmeric
Ayurvedic Supplements	• Neem Guard • Raktasodhak Bati • Arogyavardhini Bati • Surakta
Diet	• Thorough cleansing of the system is essential for the treatment of boils. To begin with, the patient may fast on orange juice diluted with water in a 50:50 ratio, or adopt an exclusive diet of fresh, juicy fruits for a few days. • After the all-fruit diet, the patient should adopt a well-balanced diet with an emphasis on whole-grain cereals, raw vegetables and fresh fruits. Further periods of a juice fast or an all-fruit diet may be necessary, depending on the general health of the patient.
Lifestyle	• Warm water should be given daily during the initial juice fast or all-fruit diet. This will help cleanse the bowels. • A warm, moist compress should be applied to the tender area.

	- Another helpful treatment for boils is a daily dry massage in the morning, followed by cold sponges. Breathing exercises in fresh air and outdoor exercises are also essential for toning up the system. In case constipation is habitual, all measures should be taken to overcome it. - The person must wash their face daily before going to sleep so that bacteria do not build up on the skin during the night.
Yoga	- Sarvangasan - Vajrasan - Viparita Karani - Ardha Kurmasan

9

Bleeding Gums

Bleeding gums are one of the common conditions affecting the oral cavity. The Chinese noticed bleeding gums as early as 2500 BC. They termed the associated diseases *Ya-Kon*, which means diseases of the soft tissue surrounding the teeth. This problem continues to affect us even with several modern facilities in oral care.

Gum disease begins with plaque, a sticky film of food particles, germs and saliva. If not removed, the plaque settles on the gum line. The germs then produce toxins that make the gums red, tender, and likely to bleed while brushing the teeth. Some chronic conditions and even medications cause plaque to accumulate quickly. The purpose of daily brushing, rinsing and flossing is to clean the plaque. When not removed, plaque can harden into tartar, which builds up along the gum line and traps germs underneath. The mildest and the most common form of gum disease is gingivitis.

The primary cause of gingivitis is the bacteria that form a layer on the teeth, and if oral hygiene is poor, it forms a sticky white substance called plaque. The bacteria here proliferate faster and produce toxins that irritate the gums, leaving them swollen and red. If left untreated, they destroy the tissues connecting the gums to the tooth and eventually the tooth to the bones, causing a deep pocket attacking the bony structure. It has now progressed into what we call periodontitis, which is an irreversible form of gum disease.

Root Causes

- Poor dental hygiene
- Gingivitis
- Gum disease
- Periodontitis
- Trench mouth
- Poorly fitting dentures
- Leukaemia
- Diabetes
- Pregnancy
- Dry mouth (a dental condition)
- Vitamin deficiency
- Certain medications

Symptoms

- Bad breath
- Bleeding is usually noticed during brushing, or in the saliva while spitting
- Eating coarse food may induce bleeding

Home Remedies	With a pinch of salt and turmeric soaked in a glass of lukewarm water, make a homemade saline solution. Use this to rinse your mouth in the morning and evening. This will help increase circulation to the gums and reduce swelling. No matter how well and often a person brushes the teeth, they can't reach the areas between the teeth and below the gums. Hence, flossing should be made a habit.

Ayurvedic Supplements	- Dant Manjan Lal - Iremedadi Tel
Lifestyle	To brush teeth to gain maximum benefits: - Push the loaded brush where the tooth meets the gum (sulcus). - Use a vibrating motion (small wiggling motion) to force the bristles into the sulcus. Do not use wide circular motions. Repeat this action along the gum line for 3–5 seconds on each spot on the sides of the cheeks and tongue. - Repeat the process until both the upper and lower gum lines are clean, inside and out. Whenever necessary, spit out any build-up of toothpaste and saliva. When done, rinse the mouth with filtered water. - Do this once a day, gradually increasing to twice a day. When able to do it twice a day, do so for two weeks. After two weeks, the gums should be tough and pink-white. **Using oral irrigators** - Another important tool to have is a Waterpik system. An oral irrigator can drastically inhibit the formation of plaque and tartar. Plaque, if not removed, turns into tartar. An oral irrigator removes approximately 50 per cent of negative bacteria with each use, leaving good bacteria that are needed to fight microbes.

	• An oral irrigator is necessary to reach areas that cannot be maintained with a toothbrush and floss alone. • Massage the gums with your finger in circular motions using some oil.
Yoga	• Simhasan (without sound) • Matsyasan (prevention purpose only) • Ustrasan (prevention purpose only)

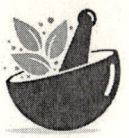

10
Breast Milk Insufficiency

Breastfeeding is an integral part of motherhood. After birth, the baby continues to receive all its nutrients from the mother through breast milk. Breastfeeding is meant to be a joyful, loving connection, and a graceful welcoming of a soul into a new body.

Nowadays, women are prone to both professional and personal stress along with poor lifestyle and food habits, which lead to various disorders.

Concept of Breastfeeding in Ayurveda

The *ahara rasa*, the essence of digestion, forms a *stanya* in the breast. Hence, stanya is termed as the *upadhatu* of rasa. The ejection of breast milk is mainly due to the suckling reflex of the baby. The first milk, colostrum, is rich in various nutrients, extremely important for newborns. It is advisable that the mother start feeding as soon as possible after the birth of the baby.

Root Causes

Primary lactation insufficiency occurs in five per cent of mothers and occurs due to inadequate glandular tissue as a result of breast abnormalities, breast or nipple surgery (which may be medically indicated or cosmetic), or other issues. Lactation insufficiency, which occurs more commonly, is usually a result of inappropriate feeding routines or use of supplements resulting in diminished milk synthesis and eventually an insufficient supply.

Suboptimal removal of milk, for example due to incorrect infant positioning and attachment, can cause this. Maternal depression, stress, or anxiety may result in a reduced response to infant feeding cues, a reduced frequency of feeds, and reduced stimulation of milk production.

Signs of Low Breast Milk

Babies may experience delayed bowel movements, decreased urinary output, jaundice, weight loss from birth, and lethargy. During breastfeeding, the baby may exhibit sleepiness or frustration at the breast, or only short periods of continuous sucking.

Management

If you wish to maintain lactation, continue nursing on demand or pump milk frequently (approximately every four hours). Pumping or expressing milk frequently between nursing sessions, and consistently when you are away from your baby, can help build your milk supply.

Healing Options

Home Remedies	- **Shatavari:** This herb, sometimes referred to as asparagus and the 'queen of herbs', is highly beneficial for mothers who are breastfeeding since it increases milk supply from mammary glands. Daily consumption of Shatavari capsules boosts the production of prolactin and corticoids, which aid in the production of breast milk, hence improving lactation and the quality of breast milk.

	• **Fennel seeds:** These are great for increasing the milk supply in nursing mothers. Fennel seeds have phytoestrogens, similar to oestrogens, which are hormones that also help in producing more milk. • **Fenugreek:** It is one of the best herbs for breastfeeding mothers to increase milk production. It also contains diosgenin and phytoestrogen. Fenugreek seeds are also loaded with galactagogue, which makes them great for mothers who wish to enhance their breast-milk supply.
Ayurvedic Supplements	• Lactone granules • Shatavari capsules • Dashmularishta
Diet	• Eating too much fast food does not provide the body the nourishment it needs. If we don't eat regularly, miss meals, and diet constantly, we essentially send our bodies into survival mode. The body thinks it is starving and shuts down unnecessary systems. A body that thinks it is starving will not have regular menstrual cycles, and having a cycle that is healthy enough to support a new life is secondary.
Lifestyle	• Try to not get agitated; be happy, and stay physically and mentally engaged.
Yoga	• Padmasan • Surya Namaskar • Bhadrasan • Shavasan

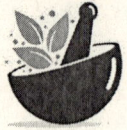

11
Constipation

Constipation is a condition of the digestive tract that restricts regular bowel movement. Improper digestion produces toxins, which find their way into the bloodstream and are then carried to all parts of the body. In chronic cases, this problem can give way to serious diseases like rheumatism, arthritis, piles, high blood pressure and even cancer. It is the root cause of different diseases like arthritis, spondylosis, irritable bowel syndrome (IBS) and hyperacidity.

Symptoms

- Infrequency, irregularity, or difficulty in eliminating hard faecal matter
- Coated tongue
- Foul breath
- Loss of appetite
- Headache
- Dizziness
- Dark circles under the eyes
- Depression
- Nausea
- Pimples
- Mouth ulcers
- Diarrhoea alternating with constipation
- Varicose veins
- Pain in the lumbar region
- Acidity

- Heartburn
- Insomnia

Root Causes

- Improper diet and irregular eating habits
- Insufficient intake of water and high-fibre food
- Excessive intake of animal protein
- Irritable colon
- Spastic colitis
- Emotional disturbances
- Lack of physical activity
- Paralytic or mechanical obstruction to the passage of stools

Healing Options

Home Remedies	• Hartaki (*Terminalia chebula*) • Isabgol (*Plantago ovata*) • Sennaleaves (*Cassia angustifolia*) • Nisoth (*Ipomoea turpethum*)
Ayurvedic Supplements	• Kabzhar • Triphala Churna • Panchasakar Churna • Gut Relief
Diet	• Avoid white flour, rice, bread, pulses, cakes, pastries, biscuits, cheese, white sugar and hard-boiled eggs. • Take the following unrefined food: **Whole-grain cereals:** Wheat **Green vegetables:** Spinach, broccoli **Fruits:** Aegle, pear, guava, grapes, orange, papaya and fig **Dairy:** Milk, clarified butter, cream • Drink at least 2.5 to 3 litres of water daily.

| Lifestyle | - Attend the call of nature regularly.
- Indulge in active physical activities or outdoor games, such as brisk walking, swimming and exercising. |
|---|---|
| Yoga | - Dhanurasan
- Yogamudra
- Vajrasan
- Ustrasan
- Pawanmuktasan |

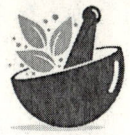

12
Common Cough

The common cough is a catarrhal and inflammatory condition of the upper respiratory tract caused by a viral, allergic or mixed infection. In Ayurveda it is known as *pratishyaya*, mainly due to the vitiation of kapha.

Symptoms

Due to the vitiation of kapha, the upper respiratory tract is inflamed and congested. Some common symptoms are sneezing, coughing, runny nose, heaviness in the head, followed by inflammation of the mucous membrane of the nose, body aches, chills and loss of appetite.

Root Causes

Allergens, viruses and bacteria are the common causative factors of this disease. A cough may be caused by the inflammation of the larynx or pharynx and develop in the chest due to changes in the weather. The real cause of this disorder is the clogging of the bronchial tubes with waste matter. The reason for the higher incidence of cough during winter than in other seasons is because of the intake of catarrh-forming food such as white bread, meat, sugar, porridge, puddings and pies. Hay fever, flu and sinusitis are the associated causes of this disease.

According to Ayurveda, pratishyaya is classified into four types—*vataj*, *pittaj*, *kaphaj* and *tridoshaj*. In vataj, there is a pain in the sinus cavity with sneezing. Pittaj is characterized by fever and in kaphaj, there is a whitish secretion and dull headache.

Healing Options

Home Remedies	• Vasaka • Garlic • Ginger • Basil
Ayurvedic Supplements	• Chyawanprash • Kasamrit Herbal • Dr Honey Syrup • Sitopladi Churna • Kantaravavaleha • Eladi Bati • Kas Bati • Talisadi Churna • Laxmivilas Ras (Naradiya) • Prawal Pishti
Diet	• In case of severe cold, cough and fever, the patient should abstain from solid food and drink only fruit and vegetable juices diluted with water. After this, the patient should adopt an all-fruit diet for 2–3 days. • Take three meals a day of fresh fruits such as apples, pears, grapes, oranges, pineapples, peaches and melons. • Unsweetened lemon water or cold or hot plain water may be given. After the all-fruit diet, the patient can gradually embark upon a well-balanced diet, with emphasis on whole-grain cereals, raw or lightly cooked vegetables, and fresh fruits.

	• The patient should avoid soft drinks, candies, ice creams and food products made from sugar and white flour.
Yoga	• Salvasan • Bhujangasan • Dhanurasan • Sasangasan • Kapalabhati

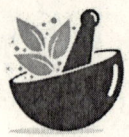

13
Colitis: Inflammation of the Colon

Colitis is caused by the prolonged irritation and inflammation of the delicate membrane lining the walls of the colon. Chronic ulcerative colitis is a severe inflammation of the colon in which ulcers form on the walls of the colon.

Symptoms

Colitis usually begins in the lower part of the colon and spreads upwards. The first symptom of the trouble is an increased urge to move the bowel, followed by cramps in the abdomen and sometimes bloody mucus in the stool. As the disease spreads upwards, the stools turn watery and more frequent, followed by rectal straining. The patient is usually malnourished and may be severely underweight.

Root Causes

One of the causes of colitis is chronic constipation and the excessive use of purgative. Constipation causes an accumulation of hard faecal matter, which is never properly eliminated. Purgatives used as a cure only increase the irritation. Often colitis results from poorly-digested roughage, especially cereals and carbohydrates, which causes bowel irritation. Other causes of the disease are an allergic sensitivity to certain food, the intake of antibiotics, and severe stress.

Healing Options

Home Remedies	• Banana • Tender coconut • Rice • Wheatgrass
Ayurvedic Supplements	• Amoebica • Isabael (H) • Chitrakadi Bati • Bhuwaneshwar Ras • Kutjarishta • Kutaj Ghanbati
Diet	• Diet plays an important role in the treatment of colitis. It is advisable to be on a juice fast for five days. In most cases of ulcerative colitis, papaya juice, raw cabbage juice and carrot juice are especially beneficial. Citrus juice should be avoided. Milk and milk products should be strictly avoided. • After the juice fast, the patient should gradually adopt small, frequent meals of soft-cooked or steamed vegetables, rice, porridge, dalia and fruits like banana and papaya. Yoghurt and homemade cottage cheese are also beneficial. All food must be eaten slowly and chewed thoroughly.
Lifestyle	During the first five days of the juice fast, the bowels should be cleaned daily after drinking warm water. Having a buttermilk enema twice a week is also soothing and helps reinstating useful bacteria in the colon. Complete bed rest is very important. The patient should eliminate all causes of tension and face the discomfort with patience.

| **Yoga** | • Vajrasan
• Pawanmuktasan
• Sarvangasan
• Ardha Kurmasan
• Ustrasan |
|---|---|

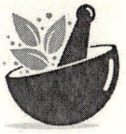

14
Cystitis (Inflammation of the Urinary Bladder)

The term 'cystitis' refers to an inflammation of the urinary bladder. The recurrence of cystitis may in some cases be associated with kidney disease.

Symptoms

The patient suffering from cystitis complains of an almost continual urge to urinate and a burning sensation while passing urine. There may be a feeling of pain in the pelvis and lower abdomen, and the urine may become thick, dark and stringy. It may have an unpleasant smell and contain blood or pus. Pain in the lower back may also be felt in certain cases. At an acute stage, there may be a rise in body temperature. In chronic cystitis, the symptoms are similar but generally less severe and long-lasting, and without fever.

Root Causes

Cystitis can be caused by an infection in other parts connected to or adjacent to the bladder, such as the kidneys, urethra, vagina or prostate gland. There may be irritation and inflammation in the bladder if urine is retained for an unduly long time. Cystitis may also result from acute constipation. Other conditions like an infected kidney, stones in the kidneys or bladder, or an enlarged prostate may also lead to this disorder or an overactive and underactive bladder (neurogenic bladder).

Healing Options

Home Remedies	• Cucumber juice • Radish leaves • Spinach • Sandalwood oil • Coriander powder
Ayurvedic Supplements	• Chandraprabha Bati • Chandanasava • Chandan Tel
Diet	• At the onset of acute cystitis, it is essential to stop eating all solid food immediately. • In case of fever, the patient should take only liquid food like fruit juices, soups, barley water and boiled vegetables. After the fever is over, the patient should take non-spicy food for a few days and then gradually embark upon all types of food.
Lifestyle	• During the first 3–4 days of acute cystitis, when the patient is on a liquid diet, it is advisable to rest and stay warm. • The pain can be relieved by immersing the pelvis in hot water. Alternatively, heat can be applied to the abdomen with a towel wrung out in hot water and covering it with a dry towel to retain warmth. The treatment may be continued for 3–4 days by which time the inflammation should have subsided and the temperature returned to normal.
Yoga	• Pranayam • Padmasan • Bhadrasan (prevention purpose) • Supta Bhadrasan (prevention purpose) • Janushirasan (prevention purpose)

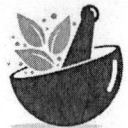

15

Cataract

The word 'cataract' signifies an opacity, which develops in the crystalline lens of the eye or its envelope, as a result of which the vision in the affected person is lost partially or completely.

Whenever an individual indulges in unwholesome activities like excessive alcohol consumption and strains his or her vision, the bodily doshas get vitiated. At first the quality of vision is impaired, then the transparency of the vision zone becomes hazy and ultimately opaque. This opacity of the visual area is known as *linganash*, the Ayurvedic name for cataract.

Classification

- Senile cataract occurs as a natural phenomenon due to ageing.
- Congenital cataract is a genetic disorder that occurs in newborn babies.
- Traumatic cataract causes opacity of the lens as a result of trauma to the eyes.
- Secondary cataract occurs in diabetic patients.

Root Causes

Cataract develops due to several reasons, including long-time ultraviolet radiation exposure, and secondarily from diseases like diabetes or simply due to advanced age.

Prevention

- UV-protection sunglass
- Antioxidant food supplements

Healing Options

Home Remedies	• Guduchi (*Tinospora cordifolia*) • Daruhaldi (*Berberis aristata*) • Amla (*Emblica officinalis*) • Baheda (*Terminalia belerica*) • Lodhra (*Symplocos racemosa*) • Shatavari (*Asparagus racemosus*)
Ayurvedic Supplements	• Saptamrit lauh • Mahatriphala Ghrit • Giloy Satwa
Diet	• Take green vegetables. • Eat fruits rich in beta-carotene, like carrot and amla. • Avoid too much salt. • Use *sendha namak* (rock salt) for cooking.
Lifestyle	• Protect your eyes from UV radiation. • Rinse eyes with triphala-soaked water or rose water.
Yoga	• Sideways and rotational viewing • Preliminary nasikagra drishti (nose-tip gazing) • Sarvangasan (for prevention purpose only) • Viparita Karani (for prevention purpose only) • Pasahastasan (for prevention purpose only)

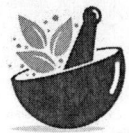

16

Cervical Spondylosis

A specific form of arthritis that affects the vertebrae is known as spondylosis. It occurs frequently in the cervical vertebrae. The spines of most people above the age of 50 have a certain degree of osteoarthritic changes. However, they seldom cause acute symptoms.

Certain precipitating factors like trauma, incorrect body posture, pressure while sleeping and excessive intake of sour food usually cause this condition. In Ayurveda it is known as *griva sandhigata vata*.

Pain in the back of the neck, shoulders and arms, stiffness of the neck and even paraplegia occur due to this condition. The movement of the spine generally aggravates the neck pain. It is often associated with memory loss and sleeplessness.

Treatment

Any external massage is not of much use. Rigorous massage with too much pressure is harmful to the patient. Only a gentle massage over the muscles of the neck and shoulder joints should be applied and for this purpose, mahanarayan oil is best suited. This gentle massage can be given two to three times a day. In the winter season, this medicated oil should be gently warmed before application.

Guggul (gum resin) extracted from the plant is the best medicine for the treatment of this condition. Ayurvedic physicians, for the treatment of this condition, popularly use a compound preparation named singhanada guggul. It is given in a dose of one to two tablets, twice a day. Usually, hot water or hot milk is given to the patient after the administration of this medicine. This medicine has a slight laxative effect. For the patient to recover from this ailment, the bowel should move clearly and regularly. In patients without constipation, this medicine should be given in a dose of two tablets and for patients suffering from constipation, the dose should be four tablets.

At night, some medicines should be given to the patients which will act as a purgative. Triphala powder is the best medicine for this purpose. One teaspoonful of triphala should be given to the patient, mixed with a cup of warm milk and one spoonful of sugar. If stools become regular with the intake of singhanada guggul, the triphala powder should be given only twice a week, otherwise it can be given every day.

According to the severity of the disease, hot fomentation on the vertebrae of the neck is very useful. Keep about 500 g of salt in a piece of cloth and warm it on a frying pan till it becomes tolerably hot. Apply this over the neck of the patient. Care should be taken that it is not too hot. In this case, it may cause burns. Sometimes, patients suffering from cervical spondylosis develop some anaesthetic patches on the back, neck, shoulders and arms because of the pressure from the nervous system. The patient is therefore unable to feel the quantum of heat applied during fomentation.

It should be the responsibility of the carer to examine the heat of the bolus before applying it to the affected parts. This fomentation should be continued for about half an hour every day. Afterwards, the affected part should not be exposed to cold wind. In the winter season, immediately after fomentation, the affected part should be covered with woollen garments. In other seasons, the affected part should be covered with cotton garments. It is convenient to take the fomentation before bedtime. The patient should then go to sleep to avoid the risk of exposure.

Healing Options

Ayurvedic Supplements	- Arth oil - Arth Plus - Rumartho Gold - Rhuma oil - Trayadanga Guggulu - Mahanarayan oil
Diet	- Sour things, especially curd, are strictly prohibited. - Fried things, pulses and various preparations of pulses are also contraindicated in this condition. - Bitter vegetables like drumstick, neem flowers and bitter gourd are useful. - Wheat is better than rice for the patient. They should, however, avoid taking refined wheat or *maida* and *suji*. To some extent, they cause constipation and do not help the patient to recover.
Lifestyle	- Exposure to cold, cold baths and any rigorous exercise of the neck muscles, including pressure, are bad for patients. - While reading and writing, one should maintain a comfortable posture. - A morning walk gives some relief to the patients, but if it is cold outside, they should always use a woollen scarf around the neck while going out of the house.
Yoga	- Abhayasan - Setu Bandhasan - Jyestikasan

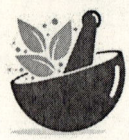

17

Chickenpox (*Laghu Masurika*)

Chickenpox is an acute and contagious disease, common in children, particularly between the ages of 1 and 10 years. Though the disease has a superficial resemblance to smallpox, it is an entirely different and less severe disease.

However, the good news is that chickenpox is a common illness in children and most people get better by just resting, like you do with a cold or the flu. The good news is that thanks to the chickenpox vaccine, many children don't get chickenpox at all. Children who do get it, if they were vaccinated, often get less severe cases, which means that they get better. Chickenpox can be prevented by getting vaccinated.

Symptoms

The disease starts with a slight fever and pain in the back and legs. There may be chills, and within 24 hours of its onset, small red papules appear on the back and chest, and sometimes on the forehead too.

A rash usually begins on the body and face and later spreads to the scalp and limbs. It may also spread to the mucous membranes, especially in the mouth and on the genitals. The rash is often itchy.

It begins as small red spots that turn into blisters within a couple of hours. After one or two days, the blisters develop scabs. New blisters may appear after three to six days.

The number of blisters differs greatly from person to person.

The infected person may have a fever. These symptoms are mild in young children.

Chickenpox lasts 7 to 10 days in children and longer in adults. Adults take longer to recover. They are also more likely to suffer more complications than children.

Root Causes

Chickenpox is caused by a virus called varicella-zoster. It may start out seeming like a cold—you might have a runny or stuffy nose, sneezing and cough. About one or two days later, the rash begins to appear, often in bunches of spots on the chest and face. From there, it can spread quickly over the entire body; sometimes the rash is even on the person's ears and mouth. The number of pockmarks is different for everyone. Some people get just a few bumps, others are covered from head to toe.

Ayurvedic Supplements	<ul><li>Neem Guard</li><li>Neem oil</li><li>Giloy Satva</li><li>Swarnamakshika Bhasma</li></ul>
Diet	<ul><li>The patient may be kept on a normal diet depending on the appetite, which is affected in some cases of fever. Hard-to-digest food should be avoided. Purgatives should also be avoided.</li><li>One capsule of Neem Guard, twice daily after a meal</li><li>Swarnamakshika Bhasma (125 mg), twice daily before breakfast and evening snacks</li><li>Haridra Khand (one teaspoon), twice daily after breakfast and dinner</li><li>Giloy Satva (250 mg), twice daily before lunch and dinner</li></ul>

Application	Sandalwood paste is to be applied to the affected area.
Lifestyle	- The infected person is contagious until new blisters have stopped appearing and all the blisters have scabs. Affected persons should stay at home while they are infectious. - Avoid scratching the blisters to avoid the risk of an infection. Cut the nails short or have the patient wear gloves. - A natural remedy is Swarnamakshika Bhasma (120 mg), taken morning and evening with a decoction of Kanchnar tree bark. - Haridra Churna (1 g) can be taken with the juice of bitter ground leaves at noon and night.
Yoga	- Vajrasan (for prevention purpose only) - Dhanurasan (for prevention purpose only) - Ustrasan (for prevention purpose only)

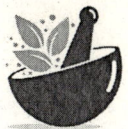

18

Cramps

Cramps are extremely common. Almost everyone (one estimate is about 95 per cent) experiences a cramp at some time in their life. Cramps are common in adults and become increasingly frequent with ageing. Children also experience cramps.

Cramping can be experienced in muscles under our voluntary control (skeletal muscles). Cramps felt in the extremities, especially the legs and feet, and most particularly the calf (charley horse), are common. The involuntary muscles of the various organs (uterus, walls of the blood vessels, intestinal tract, biliary and urinary passages and bronchial tree) are also subject to cramps.

The most commonly affected muscle groups are:

- Back of the lower leg or calf
- Back of the thigh (hamstrings)
- Front of the thigh (quadriceps)
- Feet, hands, arms and abdomen

Causes

Cramps are related to poor flexibility, muscle fatigue, or doing a new activity. Other factors associated with muscle cramps include exercising in extreme heat, dehydration and electrolyte imbalance. Cramps are more common during exercise in the heat because sweat contains fluids as well as electrolytes (salt, potassium, magnesium and calcium). They are most common in the elderly and in patients who take diuretics (a medicine that removes excess salt and water).

Primary Prevention

- Improve fitness and avoid muscle fatigue.
- Stretch regularly after exercise and warm up before exercise.
- Stretch the calf muscle in a standing position with both feet pointing forwards, and straighten the rear leg.
- Stretch the hamstring muscle. Sit down with one leg bent and one leg straight; the foot is upright and the toes and ankles are relaxed. Lean forwards slightly and touch the foot of the straight leg (repeat with the other leg).
- Stretch the quadriceps muscle. While standing, hold the upper part of the foot with the other hand and gently pull the heel towards the buttocks (repeat with the other leg).

Healing Options

Ayurvedic Supplements	- Arth Plus - Arth Oil - Rumartho Gold - Sinhanad guggulu - Mahanarayan Oil
Diet	- Patients should not be given food that aggravate vayu. - Pulses are bad for such patients. - Cold, dry, pungent and astringent food should also be avoided. - Sweet and sour food can be given to the patients in good quantity. - Garlic is helpful in such cases. - Eat bananas for natural magnesium.

| Lifestyle | • Patients should get regular massages and exercises. They should not expose themselves to cold wind or rain.
• Fasting, exercising beyond one's strength, staying awake at night, suppressing natural urges, worrying, anxiety and anger are some of the important causes of aggravation of vayu, and these should be discouraged.
• Patients should not sleep during the daytime. |
|---|---|
| Yoga | Anti-rheumatic asanas
• Tadasan
• Ardha Kati Chakrasan
• Trikonasan |

19
Conjunctivitis

The conjunctiva is a mucous membrane that extends from under the surface of the eyelids and stretches to the anterior part of the eyeball. An infection or inflammation of the conjunctiva is known as conjunctivitis.

If the three bodily doshas get vitiated by causative factors, they affect the thin layer covering the eyes, thereby causing *abhishyanda*, a painful condition of the eyes and characterized by profuse discharge there.

Root Causes

Infective conjunctivitis: This is due to infection of the conjunctiva by microbial agents like bacteria, viruses, etc.

Allergic conjunctivitis: This is due to a hypersensitive reaction of the conjunctiva to non-specific agents like dust, smoke, pollen, etc.

Symptoms

- Discomfort and foreign-body sensation in the eyes
- Redness of the eyes
- Photophobia, that is, difficulty tolerating light
- Sticking together of the eyelid margins due to profuse discharge

Healing Options

Home Remedies	• Guduchi (*Tinospora cordifolia*) • Amla (*Emblica officinalis*) • Haritaki (*Terminalia chebula*) • Baheda (*Terminalia belerica*) • Nirmali (*Strychnos potatorum*)
Ayurvedic Supplements	• Saptamrit Lauh • Mahatriphala Ghrit • Arogyavardhini Bati • Giloy Satva
Diet	• Pungent and sour food like spices, pickles and curd are contraindicated. • Avoid food that causes constipation and nasal congestion. • Fried food is not helpful. • Cow's ghee is considered very useful.
Lifestyle	• Ensure isolation and avoidance of the causative factors. • Avoid sun exposure; protect eyes with sunglasses • Wash eyes at regular intervals with cold water or rose water. • Avoid viewing television or running a computer for a long time.
Yoga	• Pranayam • Padmasan • Meditation • Padahastasan (prevention purpose) • Sarvangasan (prevention purpose) • Parivrtaa Trikonasan (prevention purpose)

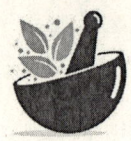

20
Diabetes Mellitus

Termed *madhumeha* in Ayurveda, its incidence is higher among the older and the obese. Originating from an absolute or relative lack of insulin, it gives way to abnormalities in the metabolism of carbohydrates, proteins and fat in the body. It is characterized by abnormally high levels of blood glucose and its subsequent excretion through urine.

Root Causes

- Overeating and consequent obesity
- Excessive intake of sugar and refined carbohydrates
- Overloading of proteins and fats, which get converted into sugar if taken in excess
- Excessive tension, worry, anxiety and grief
- Hereditary factors

Symptoms

- Constant feeling of hunger and thirst
- Weight loss
- Quick exhaustion, drowsiness and low sex drive
- Possible anaemia, constipation, itching around genital organs, heart palpitations
- Slow healing of wounds

Healing Options

| Home Remedies | - Neem (*Azadirachta indica*)
- Gurmar leaves (*Gymnema sylvestrae*)
- Karela (*Momordica charantia*)
- Nayantatra (*Vinca rosa*) |
|---|---|
| **Ayurvedic Supplements** | - Diabet Guard capsules
- Dia-fix juice
- Madhumehari granules
- Shilajit tablets |
| **Diet** | - Avoid sugar in any form. Rice, potatoes, bananas, cereals and fruits contain high sugar content.
- Do away with fatty food.
- Go for the following low-calorie, low-fat alkaline diet and high-quality natural food:
  Seeds: Purslane seeds, bitter gourd and fenugreek seeds
  Vegetables: Bitter gourd, string beans, cucumber, onion and garlic
  Fruits: Indian gooseberry, jambul fruit, grapefruit
  Grains: Bengal gram, black gram
  Dairy products: Homemade cottage cheese and various forms of soured milk, such as curd and buttermilk
- Emphasis should be on raw vegetables and herbs, as they play a part in stimulating the pancreas and enhancing insulin production. |

Lifestyle	• Don't indulge in daytime sleep. • Avoid injuring yourself as it takes time to heal. There is a possibility of the wound becoming septic. • Take adequate eye care, as the disease in serious condition might affect the eye. • If afflicted by another disease, take prompt action as diabetes can affect the immune system. • Practise foot care.
Yoga	• Bhujangasan • Shalabhasan • Dhanurasan • Apart from daily yoga, exercises like cycling, swimming and jogging must be undertaken.

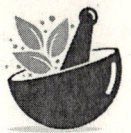

21

Dyspepsia

Dyspepsia is a word of Greek origin meaning 'indigestion' or 'difficulty in digestion'. It is a common ailment caused by dietetic problems.

Symptoms

Abdominal pain, a feeling of undue fullness after eating, heartburn, loss of appetite, nausea or vomiting, flatulence or gas are the usual symptoms of dyspepsia. Vomiting usually provides relief. Other symptoms are a foul taste in the mouth, a coated tongue and foul breath. At times, a sensation of strangling in the throat is experienced. In most cases of indigestion, patients suffer from constipation.

Root Causes

The main causes of dyspepsia are overeating, eating wrong food combinations, eating too rapidly, and neglecting proper mastication and salivation of food.

Overeating is bad for the stomach, liver and kidneys, and makes bowels harder. When the food is putrefied, toxins are absorbed into the blood and consequently, the whole system is poisoned. Certain food, especially if it is not properly cooked, cause dyspepsia. Other causes are intake of fried food, fatty and spicy food, excessive smoking, intake of alcohol, constipation, the habit of eating and drinking together, insomnia, emotions such as jealousy, fear and anger, and lack of exercise.

Healing Options

Home Remedies	• Lemon • Grapes • Carrot • Fenugreek
Ayurvedic Supplements	• Livgood Cap • Liverole Strong tablet and syrup • Livgood Juice • Chitrakadi Vati • Lashunadi Bati • Arogyavardhini Bati
Diet	The best way to commence treatment is to adopt a light diet of soup, fruits, juices, boiled vegetables, etc. The patient may thereafter gradually embark upon a well-balanced diet consisting of fresh fruits, raw and steamed vegetables, seeds, nuts and whole grains.
Lifestyle	Patients suffering from indigestion must always follow certain rules regarding eating—never hurry through a meal, never eat on a full stomach, and don't eat when you lack appetite.
Yoga	• Pawanmuktasan (Knee to chest pose) • Vajrasan • Padmasan (Lotus pose) • Ardha Kurmasan

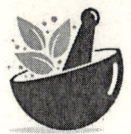

22

Dysentery

Dysentery is a term for various intestinal disorders, especially of the colon, characterized by inflammation of the mucous membranes. The types of dysentery are amoebic, bacillary, balantidium, malignant and viral.

Root Causes

- Bacterial or viral infections, infestation with protozoa or parasitic worms, and chemical irritants
- Inflammation of the rectum and large intestine, insufficient food, improper diet, drinking too much liquid with meals, overeating, wrong combinations of food, stimulating food, liquor, tea, coffee, drinking impure water, unhygienic surroundings, eating fruits or vegetables that have begun to decompose, eating food that have been standing in pantries that are not well ventilated, and eating improperly refrigerated and contaminated food
- Irritated bowels, habitual constipation, and taking certain types of medicine, such as laxatives

Symptoms

- Abdominal pain, tenesmus (spasmodic contractions of the anal or vesicle sphincter with pain and persistent desire to empty the bowel or bladder, with involuntary, ineffectual straining efforts)

- Fever, loss of appetite, sleeplessness and restlessness at night
- Diarrhoea with the passage of mucus or blood
- Distended abdomen

Severe Symptoms

- Increasing fever, excessive thirst, red tongue, abdomen may appear sunken in some cases
- Bowels become relaxed and may protrude
- Passage of urine is infrequent and is accompanied by a burning sensation
- Pulse becomes slow, breathing is rapid, and generally the patient looks pale and emaciated

Do not let this condition continue. Consult a doctor for the severe symptoms.

Healing Options

Home remedies	• Babul • Arjuna • Bael fruit • Cumin seeds
Ayurvedic Supplements	• Amoebica tablets • Isabbael (H) • Lashunadi Bati • Bhuwaneshar Ras • Biswadi Churna

| Diet | - Eat a light diet.
- Use potassium broth, soya beans milk and oatmeal milk, and drink at least a pint a day of slippery elm water and barley water.
- Whole-wheat flakes can be completely dissolved in soya beans milk.
- Chew the food thoroughly before swallowing.
- See the doctor for diagnosis and treatment. |
|---|---|
| Yoga | - Pawanmuktasan
- Vajrasan with Ashwini holding
- Padahastasan
- Paschimottasan |

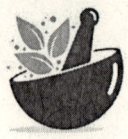

Dandruff (Scaliness of the Scalp)

The term 'dandruff' generally refers to the condition of the skin in which shiny, silvery scales separate from the scalp and collect in the hair. The condition can become troublesome when the skin gets infected.

Symptoms

While combing or brushing the hair or scratching the scalp, the dandruff falls like snowflakes and settles on the eyebrows, shoulders and clothes. This dandruff sometimes appears as lumps or crusts on the scalp. Often there is itching and the scalp may turn red from scratching.

Root Causes

The main causes of dandruff are a general impairment of health, the development of a toxic condition, mainly due to taking the wrong food, constipation and low vitality because of infectious diseases. Other factors contributing to this disorder are emotional stress, harsh shampoos, and exposure to cold and exhaustion.

Healing Options

Home Remedies	- Fenugreek seeds - Lime - Green gram powder - Snake gourd
Other Remedies	- Dandruff can be removed by massaging the hair for half an hour with curd that has been kept in the open for three days, or with a few drops of lime juice mixed with amla juice every night before going to bed. - Another measure is to dilute apple cider vinegar with an equal quantity of water and dab this on the hair with cotton wool between shampooing. Adding apple cider vinegar added to the final rinse after shampooing also helps to disperse dandruff.
Ayurvedic Supplements	- Amlaki rasayan - Guduchyadi Tel - Dhatri lauh - Kalonji oil
Diet	- Avoid spicy and greasy food because it increases dandruff. - Add more vegetables and fruits to the diet. - Take fresh food and avoid having tinned and canned food; eat more green vegetables and fruits. - Strong tea and coffee and processed food should be avoided.

Lifestyle	- The foremost consideration in the treatment of dandruff is to keep the hair and scalp clean to minimize the accumulation of dead cells. Hair should be brushed daily to improve circulation and remove flakiness.
- The most effective way to brush the hair is to bend forward from the waist, lower the head to the floor and brush from the nape of the neck to the crown. In addition, the scalp should be massaged thoroughly every day with the fingertips, working systematically over the head. This should be done immediately before or after brushing the hair. Like brushing, this stimulates blood circulation, loosens dirt and dandruff, and promotes hair growth.
- Exposing the hair to sunlight is also a useful measure in the treatment of dandruff. Use any herbal shampoo to cleanse the hair. You can also prepare and use herbal hair packs by mixing henna powder, curd and Ritha powder. Apply it on your head, leave it on for half an hour and wash it out with water. Then wash your head with a lime-based herbal shampoo. Lime is good for treating dandruff and also acts as a conditioner.
Yoga	- Bhujangasan
- Vajrasan
- Padahastasan
- Sarvangasan

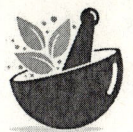

24

Depression

Depression is one of the most common emotional disorders. It may manifest in varying degrees—from feelings of slight sadness to utter misery and dejection. Depression is a very unpleasant malady and is far more difficult to cope with than a physical crisis. The mental stress and strain of day-to-day life usually lead to this disorder. There are three vital energies of the mind—the *satwa*, the *raja* and the *tama*. It is an emotional disorder caused by the aggravation of the tama.

Symptoms

- The most striking symptoms of depression are an acute sense of loss, inexplicable sadness, fatigue, and lack of interest in the world around.
- Disturbed sleep is a frequent occurrence.
- Other symptoms of depression are loss of appetite, giddiness, itching, nausea, agitation, irritability, impotence or frigidity, constipation, aches and pains all over the body, lack of concentration and indecisiveness.
- Cases of severe depression may be characterized by low body temperature, low blood pressure, hot flushes and shivering.

Root Causes

- Prolonged periods of anxiety and stress can cause depression.
- Excessive and indiscriminate use of drugs also leads to

faulty assimilation of vitamins and minerals in the body and ultimately causes depression.

Healing Options

Herbal Home Remedies	• Apple • Cashew nut • Asparagus • Cardamom • Rose
Ayurvedic Supplements	• Stress Guard • Brahmi Bati • Ashwagandharishta • Sarwatarishta
Diet	• The diet of the person suffering from depression should completely exclude tea, coffee, alcohol, cold drinks and all coloured food. • Try to take more vegetables and fresh fruits and fruit juices.
Lifestyle	• A person suffering from depression can overcome it by being more active, turning outwards, and diverting attention towards other people and things. • The pleasure of achieving something overcomes distress or misery. • Exercise also plays an important role in the treatment of depression. It not only keeps the body physically and mentally fit but also provides recreation and mental relaxation. • A person suffering from depression should practise meditation.
Yoga	• Pranayam (Basic breathing) • Meditation

25

Diarrhoea

Diarrhoea or loose and frequent evacuation of the bowels more than three times a day is a serious condition. It can be broadly categorized into two types—ordinary diarrhoea and infantile diarrhoea.

Root Causes and Symptoms

Ordinary diarrhoea

Ordinary diarrhoea may occur due to the incapacity of the bowels to cope with fatty food, ingestion of poisonous substances, certain harmful bacteria (as in cholera or typhoid fever), improper diet, ulceration of the intestines as in tuberculosis or some diseases of the liver, kidneys, lungs, or the heart. Diarrhoea may also be caused by sudden fright or shock due to the death of a loved one or worrying too much. Other causes of diarrhoea include change of climate, as with mountaineers when they reach height, change of season, as in spring or autumn, or a change to the diet to which a person is habituated.

Infantile diarrhoea

Contaminated milk or an infection of the alimentary canal may cause diarrhoea in infants. If the infant is breastfed, some of the digestive disorders of the mother may be transmitted to the child. Infantile diarrhoea may be accompanied by vomiting or gripping pain in the stomach. It is a common disorder at the time of teething. The child might cry, refuse milk, and not sleep. Care should be taken in such a condition as prolonged diarrhoea may lead to dehydration. In some cases, infantile diarrhoea starts because the child may be drinking milk from a pregnant woman.

Home Remedies

In diarrhoea of ordinary intensity, preparations made from the various parts of the babul tree are useful. A mixture of equal parts of the tender leaves of the tree with white zeera (white cumin) and black zeera (black cumin) should be administered thrice daily in doses of 12 g each. An infusion made from the bark of the tree, comprising about a couple of ounces boiled in a pint of water, should be given thrice daily. Another useful remedy is soaking 3 g of catechu (extract of acacia trees), and 4 g cinnamon for two hours in half a pint of boiling water, and giving the decoction in 10 ml doses, thrice a day.

Ayurvedic Supplements	<ul><li>Isabael (H)</li><li>Kutajghan Bati</li><li>Gangadhar Churna</li><li>Kutajrishta</li></ul>
Diet	<ul><li>A liquid or semi-liquid diet including soups of various vegetables should be taken.</li><li>Fluid loss should be compensated by intake of oral rehydration solution (ORS) to maintain electrolyte balance.</li><li>For infantile diarrhoea, the diet should consist of low-fat milk. Cow's milk or goat's milk should be given. In case cow's or goat's milk is not available, any milk should be diluted with water and consumed.</li></ul>
Yoga	<ul><li>Ardha Kurmasan</li><li>Ustrasan</li><li>Vajrasan</li></ul>

26

Epilepsy

Epilepsy may be clinically defined as a condition in which there are recurrent (two or more) unprovoked seizures. Referred to as *apasmara* in Ayurveda, epilepsy, more commonly known as the falling disease, is a serious disorder of the central nervous system that affects both children and adults alike. Afflicting infants and early teenagers the most, it is categorized into two main types—*petit mal* and *grand mal*. Depending on the dominance of the three doshas and their combined effect, it can be of four types. A fifth type, called *yoshapasmara*, is more prevalent among women.

Root Causes

- Petit mal results from a strained nervous condition.
- Grand mal is due to hereditary influences, serious shock or injury to the brain or nervous system, and diseases like meningitis and typhoid.
- Allergic reaction to certain food substances
- Circulatory disorders
- Chronic alcoholism
- Lead poisoning
- Use of cocaine
- Mental conflict
- Deficient mineral assimilation

Symptoms

- In the case of petit mal, there is a momentary loss of consciousness with no convulsions except a slight rigidity. In this case, the attack stops within a few seconds.
- Grand mal, on the other hand, has a dramatic effect. Violent convulsions accompanied by a sudden loss of consciousness, twitching of the muscles, biting of the tongue, distorted fixation of limbs, rotation of the head and deviation of the eyes last much longer.

Healing Options

Home Remedies	- Brahmi (*Bacopa monnieri*) - Shankha Pushpi (*Evolvulus alsinoides*) - Malkagni (*Celastrus paniculatus*) - Jatamansi (*Nardastachys jatamansi*)
Ayurvedic Supplements	- Brahmi Bati (with pearl and gold) - Brahmi Ghrita - Sankapushpi syrup - Ashwagandharishta
Diet	- Avoid pungent, fried and greasy food, sugar, sweets, strong tea and coffee, alcoholic beverages, condiments and pickles. - Adopt the following well-balanced diet: **Seeds:** Alfalfa seeds **Vitamin B6:** Rice, milk, brewer's yeast, cereals, legumes, carrots, peanuts, green leafy vegetables **Fruits:** Oranges, grapes, grapefruits, peaches, pears, pineapples and melons - Don't overstuff yourself. Go for frequent small meals rather than an elaborate one.

Lifestyle	• Follow a daily routine. • Try to keep stress at bay. • Keep yourself busy so that you get no time to brood. • Avoid excitement of all kinds. • Go for an invigorating head and feet massage with sesame oil, on a daily basis.
Yoga	• Meditation • Padahastan • Ardha Kurmasan • Viparita Karani with wall support

27
Eczemas

The terms 'eczema' and *vicharchika* are synonymous. Both refer to distinctive reaction patterns of the skin, which can be either acute or chronic. It is a characteristic inflammatory response of the skin.

Types of Eczemas

There are two groups of eczemas—exogenous and endogenous. While the overlap between the two groups is common, the distinction between them is critical for treatment because avoidance of carriers takes precedence over other measures in the management of exogenous eczema.

Classification of the Eczemas
Exogenous
• Irritant
• Allergic
Endogenous
• Atopic
• Seborrheic
• Discoid (nummular)
• Asteatosis
• Gravitational (stasis)
• Localized neurodermatitis
• Pompholyx (dyshidrotic)

Symptoms

- In the former, there is no secretion, whereas in the latter, fluid may be secreted from the patches, either by scratching or without it.
- Redness and swelling, usually with ill-defined margins
- Papules, vesicles and, more rarely, large blisters
- Exudation and cracking
- Scaling
- Lichenification, a dry, leathery thickening with increased skin markings, is secondary to rubbing and scratching
- Fissures and scratch marks
- Pigmentation

Healing Options

Herbal Remedies	• Babul • Butea • Linseed • Madhuca
Ayurvedic Supplements	• Neem Guard • Surakta • Raktosodhak Bati • Gandhak Rasayan • Khadirarishta
Diet	• Salt intake should be reduced. • Sour food, including pickles and curd, should be strictly avoided. • Bitter and neem flowers are useful. • Turmeric is perhaps the best as it can be applied externally.

Lifestyle	• Patients must clean the affected part(s) with water boiled with neem bark. • After cleaning, the paste of the bark should be applied over it and allowed to dry. • Avoid having spicy and oily food. • Patients need to avoid hot and humid temperatures and avoid wearing tight clothing.
Yoga	• Pranayam • Sarbangasan • Shirshasan • Padahastasan • Vajrasan • Sarvangasan

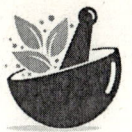

28
Enlarged Prostate

In men, the prostate gland usually starts to enlarge after the age of 40 or in middle age. This condition is called benign prostatic hyperplasia (BPH).

The prostate gland, which is normally about the size and shape of a walnut, wraps around the urethra between the pubic bone and the rectum, below the bladder. In the early stage of prostate enlargement, the bladder muscle forces urine through the narrowed urethra by contracting more powerfully. As a result, the bladder muscle becomes thicker and more sensitive, causing the urge to urinate more often.

The prostate gland secretes a fluid that is discharged with the sperm and provides nutrition and lubrication to semen. The gland itself surrounds the urethra, which is the tube that carries urine from the bladder out through the tip of the penis. As the prostate grows larger, it may press on the urethra. This narrowing of the urethra can cause some men with prostate enlargement to have trouble with urination. Prostate enlargement may be the most common health problem in men older than 60 years. Prostate cancer is the most common type of cancer in elderly males.

Symptoms

Men with an enlarged prostate usually have no symptoms. Common symptoms may include:

- Difficulty urinating
- Dribbling of urine, especially after urinating

- Feeling unable to empty the bladder
- Leaking of urine
- Frequent urination and a strong and sudden urge to urinate, especially at night
- Blood in the urine

Healing Options

Home Remedies	- Avoid drinking more liquids after 6 p.m. to reduce the need to urinate frequently at night. - Drink one cup of coriander water twice daily. - Drink eight glasses of water a day to prevent bacteria from accumulating in the bladder. - Drink cranberry juice four times a day to increase the acidity of the urine.
Ayurvedic Supplements	- Prosguard capsule - Prostaid tab - Gokshuradi Guggulu - Chandraprabha Bati - Shilajeet tablets or capsules
Diet	- Hot spices are to be strictly avoided. - The patient should be given as much water as possible. - Fresh lemon juice, coconut water, orange juice, sugarcane juice and pineapple juice are extremely useful in this condition. - The patient should be given fruits like apples, grapes, peaches and plums in good quantity.

Lifestyle	The patient should avoid exposure to sunlight or heat. Excessive perspiration removes a lot of water from the body, causing the urine to become concentrated. When the concentrated urine passes through the urinary tract, it causes irritation and a burning sensation.
Yoga	• Gomukhasan • Janushirasan • Sarvangasan

Flatulence

Flatulence is the distension of the stomach and intestines because of excess gas in the system. It is called *adhmana* in Ayurveda.

Symptoms

- Loss of appetite
- Indigestion
- Breathlessness
- Headache
- Sleeplessness

Root Causes

- Swallowing of air
- Faulty dietary habits such as eating too fast or eating spicy food
- Stress and anxiety
- Hyper-salivation due to gastritis
- Reflex from angina or chronic cholecystitis
- Fermentation in the gastrointestinal tract due to inadequately cooked starchy food
- Deficiency of *pachaka pitta* or disturbance of *samana vata*

Healing Options

Herbs	• Ginger (*Zingiber officinale*)
	• Hing (*Asofoetida*)
Ayurvedic Supplements	• Digest Guard Juice
	• Gaisantak Bati
	• Hingwastak Churna
	• Aquagest
	• Sankha Vati
Diet	• Avoid pulses, beans and fatty food.
	• Eat plenty of curd and buttermilk.
Lifestyle	• Take rest after having a full meal.
	• Drive your worries away.
Yoga	• Mayurasan (Peacock pose)
	• Pawanmuktasan (Knee-to-chest pose)
	• Leg raises
	• Ardha Kurmasan
	• Dhanurasan

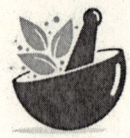

30

Fatigue

Almost everyone works long hours on certain occasions, sacrificing rest and sleep. This may cause temporary fatigue.

Symptoms

Fatigue refers to a feeling of tiredness or weariness. It can be temporary or chronic. This condition can be remedied by taking adequate rest. Chronic or continuous fatigue is, however, a serious problem that requires a comprehensive plan of treatment.

Root Causes

The main cause of fatigue in Ayurveda is an imbalance of the three doshas. A specific character trait, compulsiveness, can lead to fatigue. Many people constantly feel that they cannot rest until they have done everything that needs to be done at once. They are usually tense and cannot relax unless they complete the whole job, no matter how tired they may be.

The main cause of fatigue is lowered vitality or a lack of energy due to wrong eating habits. The habitual use of refined food, such as white sugar, refined cereals, white flour products, and processed food has adverse effects on the process in general. Certain physical and mental conditions also lead to fatigue. These include anaemia, intestinal worms, low blood pressure, low blood sugar, infections in the body, liver damage, food and drug allergies, insomnia, mental tension and unresolved emotional issues.

Healing Options

Home Remedies	• The person suffering from fatigue should eat nutritious food that provides energy to the body. Cereal grains in their natural state relieve fatigue and provide energy. These cereals are corn, wheat, rye and maize. • Vitamin B • Dates • Lemon balm
Ayurvedic Supplements	• Zest Men • Zest Women • Keshari Kalp • Musli pak • Drakshasava (Special) • Ashwagandha capsules • Shilajeet capsules
Diet	Nutritional measures are most vital in the treatment of fatigue. Studies reveal that people who eat snacks between meals suffer less from fatigue and nervousness, think more clearly, and are more efficient than those who eat only three meals daily. These snacks should consist of fresh or dried fruits, fruit or vegetable juices, raw vegetables, or small sandwiches of whole-grain bread. These snacks should be light, and less food should be consumed at regular meals. The snacks should also be taken at specified times such as 11 a.m. or 4 p.m.

Lifestyle	- *Ahara* (diet), *nidra* (sleep) and *brahmacharya* (daily routine) are the three pillars of Ayurveda. These should be properly maintained. - Chronic fatigue caused by poor circulation can be remedied by daily physical exercise. It helps relieve tension, bring a degree of freshness, renew energy and induce sleep. - Massages, gradually increasing cold applications, or alternating hot and cold baths stimulate the muscles to new activity and thus alleviate fatigue.
Yoga	- Pranayam (Basic breathing) - Sarvangasan (Shoulder stand) - Padmasan - Ardha Chandrasan - Parivrtaa Trikonasan (Twisted triangle pose)

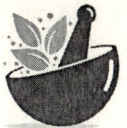

31

Fever

Fever refers to a condition of the body in which the temperature rises above normal. It is characterized by a disturbance in the normal functioning of the systems. It is a common ailment which occurs both in children and adults.

The average temperature of a healthy body ranges between 98.4°F and 99.5°F. It is liable to marginal variations, depending on the intake of food and the amount of exercise. The body temperature of a person is lowest between 1:30 a.m. and 7 a.m., and highest between 4 p.m. and 9 p.m.

Symptoms

Fever generally begins with slight shivering, pain in the head and various parts of the body, thirst and lassitude. The flow of urine is scanty. As the fever rises, the pulse and respiration become faster. Finally, there is profuse sweating, copious flow of concentrated urine, and general relief of symptoms.

Root Causes

The term 'fever' has a very wide application. It is the symptom of the body's fight against an infection. It is one of the most common features of several diseases. In many cases, it is a secondary symptom of the disordered state of the body with which it is associated. The real cause of all fevers, including common fever, however, is the accumulation of morbid matter in the system due to wrong feeding habits and unhygienic living conditions. Fever is thus a natural attempt of the body to rid itself of toxic matter.

Home Remedies	- Holy basil - Fenugreek - Saffron - Raisins - Apricot - Grapefruit - Orange - Bloodworm - *Sonthi* (Dry ginger) - Coriander
Ayurvedic Supplements	- Mahasudarshan Churna - Mahalaxmivilas Ras Vrihat - Amritarishta - Ananda Bhairav Ras (Jwar)
Diet	- The patient should be put on a fruit juice and water diet at the beginning of the treatment. The procedure consists of drinking orange juice in a glass of warm water every two hours from 8 a.m. to 8 p.m. After the temperature has come down to normal, they should eat three meals, with an emphasis on fresh fruits, and raw or lightly cooked vegetables.
Lifestyle	- While the patient is on an orange-juice fast, a warm water enema should be given daily to cleanse the bowels. - Cold compresses may be applied to the head in case the temperature rises. - Complete bed rest is advisable.
Yoga	- Pawanmuktasan (for prevention purpose only) - Sarvangasan (for prevention purpose only) - Ustrasan (for prevention purpose only)

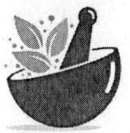

32
Female Sterility

The union of sperm and ovum, and the implantation of the foetus in the uterine wall leads to pregnancy. For its proper development, the foetus needs adequate and correct nourishment—provided through the umbilical cord. The mother, therefore, should be free of disease during the pregnancy, including throughout conception and gestation. Sterility in females is thus a result of either the defects of the ovary, uterus, fallopian tubes, or an imbalance in the hormones controlling the functions of these organs, or diseases suffered by the would-be mother.

Defects of the genitalia may be structural (organic) or functional. To correct the organic defects, surgical measures are taken. Functional defects of the organs, termed *vandhyatva* in Ayurveda and caused by the simultaneous aggravation of all three doshas, can be successfully treated with Ayurvedic medicines. Ayurveda explains *garbha sambhava samagri* (proper union of four factors, that is, periods, healthy reproductive system, healthy sperm and ovum) and *manashik abhitapa* (psychological and emotional factors) responsible for conception.

Herbal Remedies

Phala ghrita

This is an effective treatment for female sterility. Mixed with milk, phala ghrita is given to the patient in a dose of two teaspoonfuls, twice daily on an empty stomach. Vanga Bhasma is the medicine of choice for the treatment of this condition—given to the patient in a dose of 0.125 g twice daily, mixed with honey. Shilajit is one of the most effective drugs for sterility. It should be taken in a dose of one teaspoonful, twice daily.

Bala

Bala can be used both locally and internally. The root of this plant is boiled in oil and milk. It is taken with lukewarm water. This brings about a change in the mucous membrane of the genital tract that aids the effective combination of ovum and sperm in the uterus. This medicated oil is also used internally (one teaspoon) in the morning with a cup of milk.

Banyan roots

The tender roots of the banyan tree are beneficial in the treatment of female sterility when there are no organic defects or congenital deformities. The roots are dried in the shade and finely powdered. About 20 g of the powder is mixed with milk, five times the weight of the powder, and taken at night—three consecutive nights after the monthly periods are over.

Jambul leaves

An infusion of the fresh, tender leaves of the jambul tree is an excellent remedy in such cases. The infusion can be prepared by pouring 250 ml of boiling water over 20 g of fresh jambul leaves and allowing it to rest for two hours. The infusion can be taken with either two teaspoonfuls of honey or 200 ml of buttermilk.

Winter cherry

This herb is another valuable and helpful remedy. The herb should be powdered and 6 g of this powder is taken with one cup of milk for five to six nights after menstruation.

Certain nutrients, especially vitamins C and E and zinc, when supplemented into the diet have been found helpful in some cases of sterility.

Healing Options

Ayurvedic Supplements	• Vita-ex Gold Women • Sundari Kalp Forte • Shilajeet capsules • Supari Pak • Phalakalyan Ghrita • Nasta Puspantan Ras • Rajoprabatni Vati
Diet	• Women suffering from sterility should avoid alkaline and pungent food. • The person should be given fruits and sweets in large quantities.
Lifestyle	• The bowels should be cleansed by a warm water enema during the period of fasting and afterward, when necessary. • Excessive fat often results in sterility. In such cases, weight can be reduced through diet control and exercise.
Yoga	• Bhujangasan • Vajrasan • Bhadrasan • Baddhakonasan • Janushirasan

33
Gout

Gout is a painful metabolic disease characterized by recurrent attacks of acute pain and swelling, initially affecting only a single joint, usually the metatarsophalangeal joint of the big toe, and later becoming polyarticular (gradually other joints are involved and the patients experience difficulty in walking, talking and moving). Inflammation and chalky deposits in the joints because of the impairment of purine metabolism in the body are common.

In Ayurveda gout is called *vatarakta*.

Symptoms

- Pain in the toes
- Swelling
- Nausea, flatulence or vague abdominal pain
- Fever, sweating, loss of appetite, constipation, highly coloured and scanty urine

Root Causes

Impairment of digestion and metabolism because of the intake of mutually contraindicated food and non-elimination of metabolic waste products from the body are responsible for the onset of this disease.

- Hereditary factors
- Age, sex and climate are the primary factors after 40 years of age,

rare in females, and occuring commonly in temperate climates
- Excessive intake of proteins deposits urates in the tissues, and inflammatory reaction with the synovial fluid

Healing Options

| Home Remedies | - Garlic
- Guggul (*Commiphora mukul*)
- Sallaki (*Boswelia sarrata*) |
|---|---|
| Ayurvedic Supplements | - Arthplus Cap
- Kaishore Guggulu
- Panchatikta Ghrita
- Giloyghan Vati
- Guduchyadi Taila
- Balarista |
| Diet | - Freshly-harvested rice and wheat should not be given to the patient.
- Old rice, wheat, moong dal, garlic, onion, bitter gourd, papaya and green banana can be taken by the patient.
- High-fibre diet is ideal for this disease.
- Avoid high-protein diet like butter and milk, and any sour, heavy and fried food. |
| Lifestyle | - The patient should avoid intense exercises, but not sit idle either.
- Exposure to cold, wind and rain, and cold-water bath are strictly contraindicated.
- Oil massage is beneficial |
| Yoga | - Forward bends
- Padmasan
- Surya Namaskar
- Vajrasan
- Pawanmuktasan |

34
Gastritis

Gastritis is of several types, depending on the nature of inflammation and the condition of the mucous membrane and glands. Hydrochloric acid and some other digestive enzymes are secreted by the gastric glands. Inflammation of the stomach therefore results in the impairment of these secretions, leading to indigestion. In Ayurveda this condition is known as *urdhvaga amlapitta*.

Symptoms

- Loss of appetite, nausea, vomiting, headache and dizziness
- Pain and discomfort in the stomach region
- Coated tongue, foul breath, bad taste in the mouth, increased saliva, scanty urination, general feeling of uneasiness and depression
- In chronic cases, patients complain of heartburn and a feeling of fullness in the abdomen, especially after meals

Root Causes

- Habitual overeating of *virudh aahar* (incompatible food combinations) or improperly cooked food like fish and milk together (*apanva aahar*)
- Excessive intake of strong tea, coffee or alcoholic drinks
- Habitual use of large quantities of condiments and sauces
- Other causes include worry, anxiety, grief and prolonged stress
- Use of certain drugs, strong acids and caustic substances

Healing Options

| Home Remedies | - Coconut
- Rice
- Marigold
- Potato |
|---|---|
| Ayurvedic Supplements | - Aquagest
- Gaisantak Bati
- Livgood
- Gas Guard
- Diagest Guard Juice
- Kabz Care for constipation
- Acidity Guard |
| Diet | - Undertake a fast for two or three days or even more, depending on the severity of the condition.
- Drink only warm water during this period. This will give rest to the stomach and allow the toxic condition causing the inflammation to subside.
- After the acute symptoms subside, adopt an all-fruit diet for three days and eat juicy fruits like apples, pears, grapes, grapefruit, oranges, pineapple, peaches and melons.
- Thereafter, embark upon a balanced diet consisting of seeds, nuts, grains, vegetables and fruits.
- Avoid the use of alcohol, tobacco, spices, condiments, meat, red pepper, sour food, pickles, strong tea and coffee.
- Avoid sweets, pastries, rich cakes and aerated waters.
- Curd and cottage cheese should be used generously. |

Lifestyle	• Avoid stressful mental or physical work. • Try to keep anxiety, worry and anger at bay. • Take complete rest, except a walk early morning for about one kilometre, which is very useful. • Try to avoid hot drinks and food.
Yoga	• Pranayam • Padmasan • Vajrasan • Ardhakurmasan • Pavanmuktasan • Bhujangasan **Special note:** The patient should be given dry frictions and daily application of a hot compress or hot water bottle, twice a day, either on an empty stomach or two hours after meals.

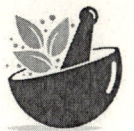

35
Gallstones

In Ayurveda the gallbladder is called *pittashaya*. However, if stones are formed in it, it is called *pittashmari*, mainly due to the vitiation of the doshas.

The gallbladder is a small pear-shaped organ that averages three to six inches in length. It lies underneath the liver on the upper right side of the abdomen. It is connected to the liver and the small intestine by small tubes called bile ducts. Bile, a greenish-brown fluid, is used by the body to digest fatty food and assists in the absorption of certain vitamins and minerals. The gallbladder serves as a reservoir for the bile. Between meals, bile accumulates and is concentrated within this organ. During meals, the gallbladder contracts and empties bile into the intestines to assist in digestion. Clinically, gallstones are called cholelithiasis.

There are two major types of gallstones:

- Cholesterol gallstones are composed mainly of cholesterol, which is made in the liver.
- Pigment gallstones are composed of calcium salts, bilirubin and other materials.

Causes

Approximately 80 per cent of all gallstones are completely asymptomatic and 'silent'. The chance that a silent gallstone will become symptomatic is two per cent each year. Women suffer from gallstones more than men. Other vulnerable groups include:

- Overweight people
- Elderly people
- Pregnant women
- Women using hormonal contraceptives and post-menopausal hormones
- People with a family history of gallstones
- People suffering from the diseases of the small intestine
- People who have recently lost weight

Symptoms

The symptoms of gallbladder disease occur when the gallstones irritate the gallbladder. The most common symptoms associated with gallstone disease include:

- Severe and intermittent pain in the right upper abdomen. This pain can spread to the chest, shoulders or back. Sometimes this pain may be mistaken for a heart attack.
- Chronic indigestion and nausea

How are gallstones identified?

Nearly all gallstones can be easily identified by an ultrasound examination. This is a simple and painless procedure in which sound waves are used to produce images of the gallbladder, bile ducts and their contents. This test is highly sensitive in identifying either gallstones or sludge within the gallbladder.

What can be done at home?

Recurrent painful attacks, if mild, can be treated with over-the-counter painkillers. Placing something warm on your stomach may be helpful (be careful not to scald the skin). The frequency of attacks may be reduced by a low-fat diet.

Can gallstones be prevented?

Recent studies suggest that people at highest risk of gallstones, like obese people undergoing weight loss, can virtually eliminate their risk of developing gallstones by taking Kanchanar Guggulu.

Healing Options

Home Remedies	<ul><li>Gokshura</li><li>Punarnavadi</li><li>Chicory</li><li>Dandelion</li><li>Olive</li><li>Sunflower oil</li></ul>
Ayurvedic Supplements	<ul><li>Livgood</li><li>Livgood Juice</li><li>Liverol Strong tablets</li><li>Gokshuradi Guggulu</li><li>Arogyavardhini Bati</li></ul>
Diet	<ul><li>Small gallstones can usually be cleared through a dietetic cure.</li><li>In the case of an acute gallbladder inflammation, the patient should fast for two or three days until the condition subsides.</li><li>Nothing but water should be taken during this period after the fast.</li><li>The patient should take fruit and vegetable juices for a few days.</li><li>Carrots, beets, grapefruit, pears, lemons or grapes may be taken in the form of juice.</li></ul>

	• Thereafter, the patient should adopt a well-balanced diet with an emphasis on raw and cooked vegetables, fruit and vegetable juices. • Yoghurt, cottage cheese and a tablespoon of olive oil twice a day should also be included in the diet.
Lifestyle	• The pain of biliary colic can be relieved with the application of hot packs or fomentation to the upper abdominal area. • A warm water enema at body temperature will help eliminate faecal accumulations in case of constipation. • Physical exercise is essential. • Surgery becomes necessary if the gallstones are very large or have been present for a long time.
Yoga	• Vajrasan • Pawanmuktasan • Padmasan • Ardha Kurmasan • Bhujangasan

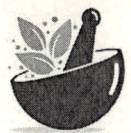

36
Goitre

This disease is characterized by the enlargement of the thyroid gland causing swelling in the front of the neck. Depending on the nature of morbidity, it is divided into several ty*pes. In* Ayurveda this is called *galaganda*.

It is usually manifested because of the lack of iodine in food and drinks. According to Ayurveda, this is caused by the aggravation of kapha and the diminution of pitta. It may be caused by both hypothyroidism and hyperthyroidism.

The enlargement of the thyroid gland in the neck becomes visible, at times becoming exceedingly large and causing difficulty in breathing and swallowing food and drinks.

Treatment

Kanchanara is the drug of choice for the treatment of goitre. The bark of this tree is given to the patient in the form of a decoction. It is administered in a dose of 30 ml twice daily on an empty stomach. Kanchanara Guggulu is popularly used for the treatment of this disease. It is given in a dose of four tablets three times a day, followed by milk or warm water.

Healing Options

Ayurvedic Supplements	• Kanchanara Guggulu • Arogyavardhini Bati • Trikatu Churna • Giloy Satwa

Diet	• Old rice, barley, moong dal, patola, drumstick, cucumber, sugarcane, juice, milk and milk products are helpful in this condition. • Sour and heavy food is contraindicated.
Lifestyle	• Exercises of the neck are useful in this condition.
Yoga	• Ustrasan (for prevention purpose only) • Sasangasan (for prevention purpose only) • Halasan (for prevention purpose)

37

Greying of Hair

Greying of hair is generally considered a sign of old age. When greying starts at a young age, it is considered as morbidity. In Ayurveda this is called *palitya*.

According to Ayurveda, excessive stress results in the greying of hair. People suffering from chronic cold and sinusitis and those who use warm water for washing their hair are more likely to be victims of this condition.

Treatments

Bhringraj and amalaki are popularly used for the treatment of this condition. A medicated oil prepared by boiling these together—mahabhringraj oil, for example—is used for massaging the head. The powder of these is also used internally in a dose of one teaspoonful, thrice daily with milk. The oil prepared from the seeds of the neem tree is used for inhalation twice a day for about a month. Along with this, the patient should be advised to take only milk as their diet.

Healing Options

Ayurvedic Supplements	• Mahabhringraj oil • Bhringarajsava • Amalaki Rasayan • Dhatri Lauha

Diet	- As far as possible, patients should take only milk and sugar. Salt should be avoided. - Sour food like yogurt is not useful. - Pungent, hot and spicy food should be avoided.
Lifestyle	- The patient should not stay awake late at night and should keep away from worry, anxiety and passion. - If suffering from cold and sinusitis, prompt and careful treatment should be given. - Hot water should never be used for washing the hair. - Cold water should always be used for bathing.
Yoga	- Padahastasan - Sarvangasan - Sasangasan

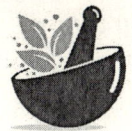

38

General Debility

General debility means a lack of strength. In Ayurveda, strength is *balam*, which is described as immunity. Charaka has used the words *Vyadhi* and *Avyadhi Kshamatwa* in this context. Those who are capable of tolerating diseases are called *Vyadhi Kshamatwa* and those who cannot tolerate diseases are called *Vayadhi Akham*, which is a symptom of general debility or general weakness and lack of strength.

Symptoms

Weakness is a very common symptom of general debility. The feeling of weakness may be subjective (feels weak but has no measurable loss of strength) or concrete measurable loss of strength. The weakness may be generalized (total body weakness) or localized to a specific area, side of the body, limb and so on.

Subjective feelings of weakness are usually generalized and associated with infectious diseases.

Weakness is particularly important when it occurs in only one area of the body.

Root Causes

- Lack of food
- Hard work
- Mental stress
- Common cold and cough

Healing Options

Herbal Remedies	- Amlaki (*Emblica officinalis*) - Satawari (*Asparagus racemosus*) - Ashwagandha (*Withania somnifera*) - Haritaki (*Terminalia chebula*)
Ayurvedic Supplements	- Zest Men - Zest Women - Musli X capsules - Amlaki Rasayan - Keshri Kalp - Chyawanprash Special - Drakshasav (Special)
Diet	- Drink more water. - If you include a certain amount of milk, cheese and eggs in your diet, you are sure to get all the nutrients you need from fats. - Eat less animal protein. - Eat more fibre-rich carbohydrates (sugar, bread, cakes and puddings). - Eat more fruits, vegetables and grains. - Use less salt and sugar in your diet. - If you drink alcohol, do so in moderation. - Eat sensibly, including plenty of fruits, vegetables, legumes and whole grains. - This type of diet should be high in immune-strengthening nutrients such as beta-carotene, vitamin E, vitamin C, vitamin B6, folic acid, zinc and selenium.

Lifestyle	• Get into the habit of exercising regularly. Avoid habits that can compromise your immune system, such as cigarette smoking, excessive alcohol intake, drug use and multiple sexual partners without appropriate protection. • Keep your chin up and try to maintain emotional stability and a positive outlook.
Yoga	• Viparita Karani • Vajrasan • Savasan

39

Gonorrhoea

Gonorrhoea is an inflammatory disease affecting the mucous membrane of the urethra in males and the vagina in females, but also spreads to other parts of the body. It is a sexually transmitted disease (STD) caused by the bacterium *Neisseria gonorrhoeae*.

Causes and Symptoms

Gonorrhoea is contagious and usually spread by sexual intercourse. However, it can also occasionally spread by using contaminated towels or clothing.

In men, this disease manifests in the form of irritation of the urethra, scalding pain on passing urine, and a viscid yellowish-white discharge. The lymph glands in the groin often become enlarged and many suppurate. The urine contains visible yellow threads of pus. When the disease continues for a long time, inflammation in the neighbouring organs may appear—the testicles, prostate gland and bladder.

At a still later stage, the inflammation of the urethra may lead to the formation of fibrous tissue around it, leading to its narrowing and difficulty urinating. The infection may spread to the various joints of the body, making them stiff.

Occasionally, general septicaemia with inflammation of the heart valves and abscesses in various parts of the body may also set in. It may also cause a severe form of conjunctivitis. In newborn babies, it may lead to total blindness. This condition is called ophthalmia neonatorum.

In females, the course and complications of the disease are somewhat different. It begins with yellow vaginal discharge, pain on passing urine, and often with inflammation of the glands situated close to the vulva (the mouth of the vagina). The most serious problem is that the inflammation may spread to the uterus, the fallopian tubes and the ovaries, causing permanent damage.

Occasionally, it may lead to peritonitis, that is, inflammation of the enveloping membrane of the abdomen, with fatal results. Many cases of continued ill health, sterility and recurring miscarriages are due to these changes.

Healing Options

Ayurvedic Supplements	• Neem Guard • Ameer Ras • Chopchinyadi churna
Diet	• Spicy food should be avoided. • More liquids should be taken.
Lifestyle	• Patients should take complete rest. • Riding horses and other forms of transport in which the hip region particularly is impacted are prohibited. • Warm water baths are indicated. • Diuretics and laxatives in case of constipation are advised. • Fluid intake should be increased, water mixed with a little milk being the chief drink.
Yoga	• Gomukhasan (for prevention purpose only) • Baddha Konasan (for prevention purpose only) • Supta Bhardasan with Ashwini Mudra (for prevention purpose only)

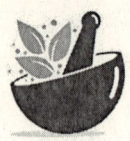

40

Hypercholesterolemia (High Cholesterol)

It is an inflammatory condition of the sebaceous glands and hair follicles that primarily affects teenagers.

Coronary heart disease is caused by high blood cholesterol. Cholesterol is essential for the human body, but some types of cholesterol can adversely affect it, causing heart attack and death. Arteriosclerosis is caused by bad cholesterol, that is, LDL cholesterol. It is a yellowish substance mainly found in the liver and in the food we consume daily.

Cholesterol is always found along with certain lipids (fats).

There are two main types of lipoproteins—low-density lipoprotein (LDL) cholesterol and high-density lipoprotein (HDL) cholesterol. HDL cholesterol is good for the human body.

Root Causes

- Obesity
- Hypothyroidism
- Diabetes
- Heredity
- Addiction to drugs or alcohol
- Stress and anxiety

Symptoms

- Angina
- Heaviness in the chest
- Heart attack
- Sudden sweating and feeling uncomfortable
- Breathlessness

Healing Options

Herbal Remedies	• Garlic (*Allium sativum*) • Gugglu (*Commiphora mukul*)
Ayurvedic Supplements	• Cholest Guard • Arjumarishta • Guggulu capsule
Diet	• Avoid excess meat, eggs, organic meat, sugar, tea or coffee, condiments, pickles, soft drinks, candies, ice creams, refined and processed food. • Eat fresh vegetables, salads, lots of lemon juice, coriander soup, mint juice and water. • Eat a low-fat diet with plenty of green salads and fruits.
Lifestyle	• Avoid sedentary habits. • Exercise daily. • Walk daily for about three kilometres.
Yoga	• Sinhasan (Lion pose) • Pranayam (Breathing exercises) • Salabhasan (Locust pose) • Vajrasan • Ardha Kurmasan • Parivrtta Trikonasan

41
Hyperacidity

It is a condition caused by the excessive secretion of hydrochloric acid in the stomach. There are several juices produced by the stomach to digest food. Hydrochloric acid is necessary to break down the food particles into their smallest form. Gastrin is the hormone responsible for the stimulation of acid secretion, whereas somatostatin suppresses acid secretion in the stomach. The excessive secretion of acid in the stomach leads to formation of ulcers.

Symptoms

- Heartburn
- Belching
- Stomach cramps
- Nausea
- Bitter taste in the mouth

Root Causes

- Irregular dietary habits
- Fried and spicy food
- Stress and anxiety
- Insomnia
- Excessive secretion of hydrochloric acid
- Loss of appetite

Healing Options

Herbal Remedies	• Mulethi • Amalaki
Ayurvedic Supplements	• Acidity Guard • Ayucid • Kamdudha Ras • Avipattikar Churna • Amlapitantak Louh
Lifestyle	• Avoid fatty, fried and spicy food, excess alcohol consumption and smoking. • Try to avoid stress.
Yoga	• Halasan (Plough pose) • Dhanurasan (Bow pose) • Pawanmuktasan • Bhujangasan • Ardha Kurmasan • Vajrasan

High Blood Pressure (Hypertension)

Regarded as the silent killer and the biggest menace of the present generation, hypertension occurs when blood pressure exceeds the systolic pressure—the highest pressure reached during each heartbeat.

Symptoms

- Pain in the back of the head and neck on waking up, which soon disappears
- Dizziness
- Palpitations
- Angina
- Frequent urination
- Nervousness
- Fatigue
- Breathing problems

Root Causes

- Stress and hectic lifestyle
- Vitiation of vata
- Smoking and excessive intake of intoxicants
- Hardening of arteries
- Obesity
- Metabolic disorders

- Excessive intake of salt
- Overeating fast food

Healing Options

Herbal Remedies	• Sarpagandha (*Rauwolfia serpentina*) • Jatamansi (*Nardostachys jatamansi*)
Ayurvedic Supplements	• Sarpagandhaghan Bati • Sarpagandha tablets • Stress Guard • BP balance juice
Diet	• Food should be consumed either raw or steamed. • The amount of oil (olive oil or mustard oil) in the food should not exceed one or two teaspoons a day. • Avoid excessive salt (not more than one teaspoon a day). • Follow the following vegetarian diet: **Vegetables:** Garlic, lemon, parsley **Fruits:** Indian gooseberry, grapefruit, watermelon **Dairy:** Milk, cottage cheese, clarified butter • Avoid alcohol and smoking • Coffee should be avoided. Tea can be taken in moderation (twice a day).
Lifestyle	• Try to get eight hours of sleep every night. • Proper rest is of primary importance. • Avoid overstraining yourself. • Don't worry! Be happy.
Yoga	• Sarvangasan (Shoulder stand) • Bhujangasan (Cobra pose) • Tadasan • Ardha Kati Chakrasan • Gomukhasan
Ayurvedic Massage	• Mahanarayan oil • Brihat Vishnu oil

43

Hair Loss

The hair is a complex and delicate part of the body. Keeping it healthy and beautiful is a challenge.

Hair is cylindrical and made of dead tissue. Damaged hair can never be fully restored to its original condition. The main factor in the growth of hair is the kind of cells that exist in the hair follicles—the growing point of the hair. Each hair strand is different from the others. Haircare products are intended to promote certain favourable conditions for the hair to reduce or eliminate properties of the hair which are regarded as undesirable.

Symptoms and Causes

Reasons for hair loss

Both men and women lose hair for similar reasons. Hair loss in men is often more dramatic and follows a specific pattern termed male pattern baldness. This loss is caused by high levels of the hormone dihydrotestosterone (DHT).

Factors for male hair loss include heredity, hormones and ageing. This may also apply to women, but to a lesser degree. Women may experience loss of hair after menopause and for two to three months after having a baby. Other contributing factors include poor diet, poor circulation, acute illness, radiation, chemotherapy, high stress, thyroid imbalance, certain drugs, coming off contraceptive pills, diabetes, high doses of vitamin A (more than 100,000 IU), sudden weight loss, high fever, iron deficiency, ringworm, some fungal infections, chemicals and hair dyes, vitamin deficiencies, and lack of proper nutrition.

Drastic or premature hair loss may be caused by:

- Stress and bodily weakness from overwork
- Dietary imbalances or nutritional deficiency
- Using abrasive shampoos, hair lacquers, dyes and bleaches
- Endocrine disorders
- Genetic factors
- Infectious diseases
- Hormonal metabolic changes in lactating women
- Nutrient and protein deficiencies in the hair cells

Modern-day problems associated with hair and scalp

For most hair-related problems, internal medicine plays a more important role than external application. In recent times, many ailments have caused hair loss. There are many problems associated with hair and scalp because of:

1. Air and water pollution
2. Use of shampoos and conditioners containing harsh chemicals
3. Use of combs and brushes in barber shops and beauty salons

Scalp problems are caused by poor immunity, or because of frequent washing with strong soaps and shampoos, excessive secretion of oil by sweat glands, and overexposure to sunlight.

Three common diseases associated with the scalp are:

- Seborrhoea
- Dandruff
- Hair loss

Healing Options

Herbal Remedies	- Bhringraj - Amla - Heena - Jaba
Ayurvedic Supplements	- Mahabhringaraj oil - Bhringaasava - Amlaki Rasayan - Amla oil
Lifestyle	- The foremost consideration in the treatment of hair loss is to keep the hair and scalp clean to minimize the accumulation of dead cells. - The hair should be brushed daily to improve circulation and remove flakiness. - The most effective way to brush hair is to bend forward from the waist and brush from the nape of the neck to the crown.
Yoga	- Vajrasan - Pawanmuktasan - Padahastan - Sarvangasan

44

Hiccups

Hiccups are characterized by the sharp inspiratory sound produced with the spasm of the glottis and diaphragm. In Ayurveda it is known as *hikka roga*. Depending upon the doshas involved in the pathogenesis of the disease, different types of symptoms are manifested.

Treatment

The ash of peacock feathers is considered to be the best therapy for the condition. It is given in a dose of 0.125 g four to six times a day, mixed with honey. Eladi bati, which contains cardamom as an important ingredient, is popularly given for the treatment of this condition. It is taken with honey to be sucked in a dose of one tablet four to six times a day.

Healing Options

Ayurvedic Supplements	• Mayur Chandrika Bhasma • Eladi Bati
Diet	• Kulatta is considered a very important herb for the treatment of this ailment. The juice or soup of this herb can be given to the patients. Old rice, patola, tender radish, lemon, goat's milk and garlic can also be given. • Fatty food, heavy and cold food, and masha (black gram) are contraindicated in this condition.

Lifestyle	• The patient should be given psychotherapy if the hiccups are caused by psychoneurotic conditions.
Yoga	• Surya Namaskar (Sun salutation) • Pranayam (Breathing exercises) • Ardha Chandrasan • Ustrasan • Setu Bandhasan

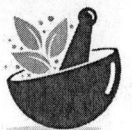

45

Haemoptysis

Spitting up blood while coughing is called haemoptysis. This is primarily caused by diseases such as tuberculosis and cancer of the lungs. In Ayurveda it is included in the group *urdhvanga rakta pitta*. The patient spits up blood while coughing. Sometimes the blood is accompanied by mucus.

Treatment

Vasaka is the drug of choice for the treatment of this condition. It is given to the patient in the form of juice in a dose of two teaspoonfuls four times a day. It is bitter and is, therefore, given to the patient mixed with honey.

Prawal Pishti, a preparation of coral, is the drug of choice for the treatment of this condition. It is given in a dose of 1 g four times a day mixed with honey.

Healing Options

Ayurvedic Supplements	• Kasamrit Herbal • Basant Malti Ras • Prawal Pishti • Giloy Satwa

Diet	- Hot and spicy things should be avoided. - The patient should be given pomegranate, amlaki, cow's milk and water. - Old rice, soup of patola, moong, masoor and meat can be given to the patient.
Lifestyle	- The patient should not exercise and take complete rest. - The patient should avoid exposure to the sun.
Yoga	- Surya Namaskar - Pranayam - Matsyasan (for prevention purpose only) - Ustrasan (for prevention purpose only) - Ardha Chakrasan (for prevention purpose only)

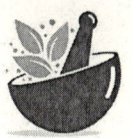

46
Heart Disease

This disease is essentially characterized by chest pain because of the increased work of the heart. It is usually relieved by rest. In most cases, the disease manifests in front of the chest and mostly above the sternum. It may spread towards the left or right side of the chest. The pain radiates towards the left side very often. It may spread to the arms, neck, jaws and the upper part of the abdomen. The left shoulder and left arm are often affected. It is commonly called heart disease.

In Ayurveda it is known as *bridroga*. It is of several types depending on the kind of pain. If the pain is acute and shifting, it is usually known as *vatika bridroga*. If it is associated with a burning sensation, it is called *paittika bridroga*. In *kaphaja bridroga*, the pain is usually very mild and associated with heaviness, nausea and cough.

Root Causes

Heart diseases are usually caused by the obstruction of the coronary arteries. These are the blood vessels that nourish the heart muscle. Since the heart muscle uses a huge amount of energy, it needs ceaseless nourishment. It naturally demands a good supply of blood. Any impairment of these blood vessels interferes with adequate blood flow to the heart muscles. If the blood flow is significantly diminished, then the heart signals pain or discomfort in the chest.

Treatment

Arjuna is the drug of choice for the treatment of this disease. The bark of this tree is used as a medicine. The powder or decoction of the bark is given to the patient during and even after the attack. The powder is given in a dose of 1 g, four times a day. If the heart disease is of the vatika type, it is mixed with ghee. If it is of the paittika type, then milk is used.

In kaphaja type of heart disease, the bark is mixed with honey or pippali powder. For the decoction, usually 30 g of the raw powder of the bark of the drug is boiled with approximately 500 ml of water and reduced to one-fourth. This is then filtered, honey or ghee is added, and given to the patient. With honey, the decoction should be cold before mixing. Ghee is mixed when the decoction is warm and is given to the patient as such.

There are many preparations of arjuna. Arjunarishta is commonly used by physicians. Six teaspoonfuls of this liquid drug are given to the patient twice daily after food with an equal quantity of water. Arjuna is boiled in cow's ghee, and this medicated ghee is given to the patient in a dose of one teaspoonful twice daily on an empty stomach, mixed with a cup of warm milk. This preparation is known as Arjuna ghrita. It should not be given to a person who is overweight. This is likely to add to the fat and may create more problems.

Other medicines used for different types of heart diseases are Hridayarnava rasa and Prabhakara vati. These medicines are available in the form of tablets. Two tablets are given to the patient, three or four times a day, depending on the seriousness of the disease.

At the time of an acute attack, Mrigamadasava is the ideal drug. It is a liquid medicine that is given to the patient in a dose of ½ to 1 teaspoonful mixed with an equal quantity of water. These medicines are to be used even after the attack has subsided. On exertion, the patient may get the attack at any time. It is therefore necessary for the patient to use the medicines mentioned above for about six months continuously.

Healing Options

Herbal Remedies	- Arjuna (*Terminalia arjuna*) - Garlic (*Allium sativum*) - Cinnamon
Ayurvedic Supplements	- Goodheart - BP balance juice - Arjunarishta - Arjun Chal Churna
Diet	- Fried food, pulses and their preparations and groundnut oil are prohibited. - Ayurvedic physicians allow using butter or ghee but not groundnut oil. - Cow's ghee, cow's milk and cow's butter are useful for the patient. Buffalo ghee and buffalo milk are not recommended. - Stimulants like tea, coffee and alcoholic drinks are harmful for such patients.
Lifestyle	- Ayurveda considers the functions of the heart and mind interlinked, as a disturbance in one affects the other. Therefore, patients with heart disease are advised to refrain from anxiety, worry and wrathful disposition. - All efforts should be made by the patient to get a good night's sleep. Even rest during the day is essential. - The patient's bowels should move regularly. If there is constipation, they are advised to drink a glass of water early in the morning and go for a walk every day.
Yoga	- Viparit Karani (for prevention purpose only) - Sarvangasan (for prevention purpose only) - Trikonasan (for prevention purpose only)

Indigestion

Not quite a disease by itself, this condition is called *agnimandya* in Ayurvedic terminology. It denotes a condition where food taken does not get digested.

Root Causes

- Aggravation of the three doshas
- Excessive intake of improper food
- Factors such as anger, anxiety and worry
- Fast eating habits
- Eating less high-fibre food

Symptoms

- Heaviness in the stomach
- Stomach pain
- Vomiting
- Nausea
- Diarrhoea
- Acidity
- Burning sensation in the chest

Healing Options

| Herbal Remedies | - Hing
- Ginger (*Zingiber officinale*)
- Lemon juice with rock salt |
|---|---|
| **Ayurvedic Supplements** | - Digest Guard
- Digest Guard Juice
- Aquagest
- Gaisantak Bati
- Agni Bardhak Bati
- Lavan Bhaskar Churna |
| **Diet** | - Take a light and low-fat diet.
- Drink plenty of water and juices, especially lemon juice mixed with a pinch of salt.
- Intake of raw garlic is beneficial. |
| **Lifestyle** | - Avoid sleeping just after having a full meal.
- Try to gain mental peace.
- Physical exercise is essential. |
| **Yoga** | - Mayurasan (Peacock pose)
- Sarvangasan (Shoulder stand)
- Pawanmuktasan
- Bhujangasan
- Ardhakurmasan |

48

Insomnia

Denoting a complete lack of sleep, insomnia has assumed alarming proportions in modern times. Sleep disturbances affect the glands and the proper secretion of hormones. There has been a manifold rise in ailments like heart diseases and high blood pressure.

Symptoms

- Sleeplessness
- Memory lapse
- Lack of concentration
- Loss of coordination
- Confusion

Root Causes

- Aggravation of vata and pitta
- Stress
- Suppressed feelings and acute bitterness
- Constipation
- Dyspepsia
- Excessive intake of tea and coffee
- Environment factors like excessive cold, heat or change in environment

Healing Options

Home Remedies	• Brahmi (*Bacopa monnieri*) • Jatamansi (*Nardostachys jatamansi*) • Ashwagandha (*Withania somnifera*) • Sarpagandha (*Rauwolfia serpentina*)
Ayurvedic Supplements	• Nightzz • Stress Guard • Brahmi Bati • Ashwagandharistha
Diet	• Go for a low-salt diet. • Avoid white flour, sugar, tea, coffee, chocolate, cold drinks, alcohol, fatty and fried food. • Take the following diet: **Vitamin B1:** Whole grain, cereals, pulses and nuts **Vegetables:** Lettuce, bottle gourd **Dairy:** Milk, curd, clarified butter **Seeds:** Aniseed
Lifestyle	• Exercise daily and walk at least one km a day. • Enjoy a stress-free life. • Cultivate a creative hobby. • Avoid meeting impossible targets. • Meditate.
Yoga	• Bhujangasana • Shavasan • Gomukhasan • Janushirasan • Ardha Kurmasan
Ayurvedic Massage	• Massage the whole body with Mahamas or Mahanarayan oil.

Immunity Disorders

Most modern diseases are caused by prolonged exposure to a combination of poor lifestyle, food habits and toxic environmental factors. Chronic stress is one of the major reasons for immune disorders.

There are two types of immunity that protect our body from any infection—innate and adaptive. Innate immunity is present at birth and provides the first barrier against microorganisms which cause infections. Adaptive immunity is the second barrier against infections and is acquired later in life via immunization. In Ayurveda, immunity is known as *byadhikshamata oja* and categorized as *par oja* and *apar oja*.

AIDS is an example of an immune disorder.

Symptoms of Weak Immunity

- Recurrent infections
- Lack of energy without any pathology
- Easily affected by diseases
- Easily tired and overstressed

Root Causes

- Microorganisms
- Genetic
- Virus
- Poor lifestyle and food habits

- Pollution
- Stress
- Metabolic disorders

Healing Options

Herbal Remedies	• Giloy (*Tinospora cordifolia*) • Neem (*Azadirachta indica*) • Amalaki (*Phyllanthis embelica*) • Aswagandha (*Withania somnifera*)
Ayurvedic Supplements	• Immune Guard • Stress Guard • Giloy Satwa (powder) • Amalaki Rasayan (powder) • Aswagandhadi churna (powder)
Diet	Patients should drink milk, buttermilk, sugarcane juice and easily digestible food.
Lifestyle	• One should follow the recognized conventions and traditions of their family and religion. • The following natural urges should not be suppressed—passing of flatus, defaecation, urination, sneezing, weeping, vomiting, breathing when fatigued, thirst, hunger and sleep.
Yoga	• Shirshasan • Meditation • Dhanurasan • Ustrasan • Sarvangasan

50
Influenza

Influenza, also known as flu, is a clinical condition caused by infection with the influenza viruses.

Symptoms

- Chills, fever, headache and severe muscular pains
- Feeling miserable and weak
- Inflammation of the nose and throat, which may spread down the windpipe to the lungs, resulting in a sore throat, cough, runny nose and watery eyes

Root Causes

- Usually occurs during the seasonal change
- Viral infections
- Affects those with a toxic and run-down condition

Healing Option

Home Remedies	- Garlic - Turmeric - Ginger - Basil
Ayurvedic Supplements	- Immune Guard - Tribhuvankirti Ras - Mahasudarshan Churna - Laxmivilas Ras (Nardiya)

| Diet | - Avoid eating heavy food; instead opt for fruit and vegetable juices.
- Take an all-fruit diet with milk.
- Avoid taking alcohol, tobacco, strong tea and coffee.
- Have lots of vegetables and fruits.
- Drink warm water. |
|---|---|
| Lifestyle | - Make sure you do not have constipation. Take an Ayurvedic laxative at night before sleeping. |
| Yoga | - Shavasan
- Yogamudra
- Tadasan
- Ardha Chandrasan
- Ustrasan |

51

Intestinal Worms

Worms are intestinal parasites that infest humans all over the world. However, they are more common in tropical and subtropical regions and prevalent during the rainy season. The eggs of the parasites are introduced into the person's system through food or water.

Symptoms

- Diarrhoea, foul breath, dark circles under the eyes, constant desire for food, restlessness at night with bad dreams, anaemia and headaches
- Roundworms cause inflammation of the intestines and lungs, nausea, vomiting, loss of weight, fever and nervousness

Root Causes

- Eating contaminated food is frequently a factor.
- Hookworms enter the human body while walking barefoot or on infected earth.
- Tapeworms are transmitted to the body through undercooked meat or food contaminated by dogs.
- The real cause of intestinal worms, however, is faulty living. The eggs of these worms can breed in the intestines if they find a suitable medium for their propagation. The medium is usually an intestinal tract clogged with morbid matter.

Healing Options

| Herbal Remedies | • Vasaka
• Coconut
• Garlic
• Papaya |
|---|---|
| Ayurvedic Supplements | • Krimighatini Bati
• Birangasava |
| Diet | • The treatment for intestinal worms should begin with diet. The patient should be kept on an exclusive fresh-fruit diet for four or five days. Thereafter, they may adopt a well-balanced light diet consisting mainly of fruits, vegetables, milk and whole-meal bread. The diet should exclude fatty food such as butter, cream, oil and all-meat food. |
| Lifestyle | • During the all-fruit or fasting period, the bowel should be cleansed daily with a warm water enema. |
| Yoga | • Vajrasan
• Pawanmuktasan
• Ardha Kurmasan
• Janushirasan |

Irregular Menstrual Periods

A normal menstrual period lasts from 2 to 7 days. The normal cycle patterns can range from 21 to 35 days. Bleeding outside the regular cycle, longer or heavier periods occurring between periods, longer than normal time between periods, or an absence of periods is called irregular uterine bleeding.

There are various causes of abnormal menstrual cycles, but the most common is hormonal imbalance. This can occur as a result of weight loss or gain, heavy exercise, stress, illness or certain medications.

Women of menstruating age may experience irregular periods. Abnormal periods are not always a cause for concern. Reasons for abnormal periods can be both normal and abnormal. The most normal reason is pregnancy.

Causes

- Stress
- New cycle, that is the irregularity experienced by young girls at the onset of their periods; their cycle can be irregular for months or years at the onset
- Eating disorders like anorexia and bulimia or simply poor diet
- Too much exercise
- Prescription and recreational drugs
- Break in routine
- Thoughts and emotions
- Sexual activity, especially when it is a new occurrence

- Anxiety about pregnancy
- Illness or physiological imbalances like thyroid disease

Treatment for Painful and Irregular Menstruation
- A piece of fresh ginger (*adrak*), ground and boiled in a cup of water. The infusion is taken thrice daily after meals along with sugar.
- Boil one teaspoon of saffron (*kesar*) in half a cup of water and let it reduce to one tablespoon. Divide this decoction into three portions and take it with equal quantities of water, thrice daily for a couple of days.
Treatment for Delayed Menstruation
- Take half a teaspoon of finely-ground cinnamon (*dalchini*) every night along with a cup of milk.
- Take a teaspoon of dried mint (pudina leaves) powder and take it with one teaspoon of honey, thrice daily.
Treatment for Excessive Menstrual Bleeding
- Grind some bael leaves into a fine paste. Take one teaspoon of warm water and drink some cold water as well.
- Boil one teaspoon of coriander (*dhania*) seeds in two cups of water until it is reduced to one cup. Add sugar to taste and drink when lukewarm. Repeat twice or thrice a day.

Healing Options

| Home Remedies | - Ashoka
- Chandan
- Lodhra
- Kamal Phool |
| --- | --- |
| Ayurvedic Supplements | - Meno Guard
- Sundari Sakhi
- Ashokarishta
- Rajaprabartini Bati |

Diet	- A good diet is important for good health. If you eat a lot of fast food, your body will not get the nourishment it needs. If you eat sporadically, miss meals and diet constantly, you essentially send your body into survival mode. The body thinks it is starving and shuts down unnecessary systems. A body that thinks it is starving will not support regular menstrual cycles. Having a cycle healthy enough to support new life is secondary.
Lifestyle	One shouldn't get agitated, but try to stay happy and keep physically and mentally engaged.
Yoga	- Bhujangasan - Sarvangasan - Ardha Chakrasan - Gomukhasan - Bhadrasan with Ashwini

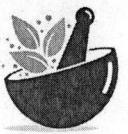

53

Jaundice and Hepatitis

The most common of all liver ailments, jaundice and hepatitis are caused by an increase in bile pigments and bilirubin in the blood, giving the skin and mucous membrane a yellow tinge. It is called *kamala* in Ayurveda.

Symptoms

- Extreme weakness
- Severe headaches
- Constipation
- Nausea
- Yellow discoloration of the eyes, tongue, skin and urine
- Dull ache in the liver region of the stomach
- Possible itching all over the body

Root Causes

- Excessive circulation of pitta (bile pigments) in the blood
- Obstruction in the bile duct or impairment of the functions of the liver or excessive destruction of the red blood cells
- Diseases such as typhoid, malaria, yellow fever and tuberculosis
- Viral infections

Healing Options

Home Remedies	• Ghritkumari (Aloe vera) • Kakmachi (*Solanum nigrum*) • Jaundice berry (*Berberis vulgaris*) • Bhumi Amla (*Phyllanthus niruri*)
Ayurvedic Supplements	• Livgood • Livgood Juice • Liverol Strong • Punarnava Mandoor • Bhumi Amla capsules • Kumari Asav
Diet	• Go for a boiled and less spicy diet. • **Vegetables**: Radish leaves, tomato, lemon • **Dry fruits**: Dried dates with almonds and cardamom • Have plenty of sugarcane juice, orange juice, bitter luffa and barley water. This improves urination, which helps eliminate excess bile pigments from the blood.
Lifestyle	• Take complete rest. • Try to stay free from anxiety and anger.
Yoga	• Matsyasan (Fish pose) • Sarvangasan • Baddhapadmasan (Hidden lotus pose) • Vajrasan • Padmasan • Savasan

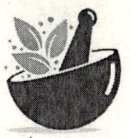

Joint and Muscle Pain

According to Ayurveda, most joint and muscle pain is caused by the aggravation of the vata dosha. It is a condition caused by accumulation of ama and aggravation of vata. This ama circulates in the entire body and deposits at weaker sites. When it is deposited in the joints and at the same time there is an aggravation of vata, it results in a disease called *amavata* that causes joint pain.

Symptoms

- The main symptom of this disease is severe pain in the affected joints. The tissues in and around the joints become inflamed and movement of the joints becomes extremely painful.
- Fever
- Immense pain and stiffness in the affected muscles, especially in the fingers, wrists, elbows, knees and ankles in the morning
- Excruciating pain and stiffness in the joints

Root Causes

- Joint injury, strain or sprain
- Previous joint injury
- Infections like viral fever, common cold, flu and bacterial infections may cause aching joints and aching muscles

Joint pain can be caused by both internal and external factors. Ama associated with vata (internal moving body air) quickly moves to different parts of the body and accumulates where circulation is sluggish or slow, such as in the hands, knees and other bone joints, filling the blood vessels with a waxy material. It is also more common in old age when vata naturally increases in the body.

Meat diet, ice creams, concentrated dairy products like aged cheese, sour cream or cheese, cold food especially during cold weather which weakens digestion, heavy cakes, pastries and candies, packaged and processed food with little fibre content are the main dietary causes.

Gas-forming vegetables and legumes create more internal air, which moves the toxins to different parts. This ama blocks tissue pores and passages, causing heaviness and weakness of the heart, which becomes the seat of the disease.

Healing Options

Ayurvedic Supplements	<ul><li>Arth Plus</li><li>Arth Oil</li><li>Rumartho Gold</li><li>Mahayograj Guggulu</li><li>Rashnadi Guggulu</li><li>Maharashnadi Kada</li></ul>
Ayurvedic Massage	<ul><li>Mahanaryan Tel</li><li>Mahamas Tel</li><li>Saindhavadi Tel</li><li>Rhuma Oil</li><li>Arth Oil</li><li>Arth Plus</li><li>Rhumartho Gold</li></ul>

Diet	• Avoid curd and sour food, pulses (except moong dal), rice, meat, fish, white bread, sugar, refined cereals, fried food, tea or coffee. • Drink potato and lemon juice. • Celery seeds and bitter gourd are beneficial.
Lifestyle	• Bowels should be cleansed daily. • Avoid damp places and exposure to cold weather. • Don't indulge in daytime sleeping. • Limit yourself to restricted exercise.
Yoga	• Tadasan • Ardha Koti Chakrasan • Padahastasan (Wide-leg pose)

Kidney Stones

Urinary stones are formed by calcium, phosphates or oxalates. The main parts of the urinary tract are the kidney, ureter, bladder and urethra. The stones are formed primarily in the kidneys and often go unnoticed for a long time. In certain circumstances, they slowly dissolve, and during this process, they become lodged in a narrow part of the tract, causing excruciating pain.

Stones are formed in the body because of vayu. It creates a type of dryness in the body because of which the chemicals start accumulating over the nucleus, which ultimately takes the shape of a stone. At times the entire kidney is filled with these stones and it becomes calcified and stops functioning.

If urine is not excreted through the kidneys, or excreted in small quantities, uraemia sets in and causes many complications. The same phenomenon takes place if a piece of stone gets lodged in the ureter or bladder.

Symptoms

The patient experiences pain in the lumbar region, which might radiate towards the genitals. This might be accompanied by fever, vomiting, loss of appetite, sleeplessness and painful urination. At times, blood may appear in the urine.

Causes

The most common cause of kidney stones is not drinking enough water. Try to drink enough water to keep the urine clear (about 8 to 10 glasses of water a day). Some people are more likely to get kidney stones because of a medical condition or family history.

Kidney stones may also be an inherited disease. If other people in your family have them, you may also have them. Some people are more susceptible to kidney stones, as heredity certainly plays a role.

The majority of kidney stones are made of calcium, and hypercalciuria (high levels of calcium in the urine) is a risk factor. The predisposition to high levels of calcium in the urine may be passed on from generation to generation.

Healing Options

Home Remedies	• Gokshura powder • Varuna powder • Shilajit powder
Ayurvedic Supplements	• Pathrina • Gokshuradi Guggulu • Varun capsules • Shilajit tablets or capsules
Diet	• The patient should not eat beans and pulses. The yellow variety of pumpkin and lady's finger should strictly not be eaten. The white variety of gourd is very useful in this condition. • Drink plenty of water.

Lifestyle	- Patients should not sit continuously for a long time after eating food. - They should either walk for a few minutes or lie down or sit on a soft cushion. - Patients should develop the habit of drinking plenty of water, which will help them to cleanse the urinary system and prevent the formation of stones.
Yoga	- Vajrasan - Paschimottanasan (Forward bend) - Ustrasan - Ardha Chandrasan - Setubandhasan

56

Leucorrhoea

This is a catarrhal discharge from the mucous membrane of the female genital tract. It is commonly known as white discharge. It may be due to pathology or due to poor health and hygiene. The vaginal discharge may vary from white to reddish or thick and viscid, with or without a foul smell, depending on the type of infections that persist. In normal cases, it may appear just before or after menstrual bleeding.

In Ayurveda this is known as *swet paradar* and believed to be caused by the aggravation or vitiation of kapha dosha.

Symptoms

- Irritability
- Digestive disturbances
- Dark circles around the eyes
- Itching in the genital region
- Stains on underwear
- Foul smell

Root Causes

- Metabolic and hormonal disturbances
- Anaemia
- Fungal infections
- Chronic amoebiasis
- Chronic constipation
- Poor hygiene

Healing Options

| Home Remedies | • Aparajita roots
• Durba juice
• Shatavari |
|---|---|
| Ayurvedic Supplements | • Lukonil tab
• Pushyanug churna
• Patrangashav |
| Diet | • Fried and spicy food should not be given to the patient.
• The patient should not be permitted to keep her stomach empty for a long time.
• She should not eat heavy, indigestible food.
• Sour food, especially pickles and curd, should be avoided.
• Intake of *supari* (betel nut) after food is both prevention and cure for this disease. |
| Lifestyle | • A brisk walk in the early morning helps in early cure.
• Sanitary and hygienic measures should be followed carefully. |
| Yoga | • Ardha Chakrasan
• Uttanasan
• Pawanmuktasan
• Dhanurasan
• Baddhakonasan
• Gomukhasan
• Viparita Karani |

Leukoderma

Leukoderma, also known as vitiligo, is a distressing skin condition. The word literally means 'white skin'. There is a gradual loss of the pigment melanin from the skin, which causes white patches. This condition does not cause any organic harm.

Symptoms

The disease usually begins with a small white spot, which later forms bigger patches. These patches are pale in the beginning, but become whiter with time due to loss of pigment. As the spot enlarges, they merge into each other and in the course of time form broad patches. In some cases, most of the body is covered with white patches.

Root Causes

The main causes of leukoderma are excessive mental stress, chronic or acute gastric disorders, impaired hepatic function, such as jaundice, worms or other parasites in the alimentary canal, typhoid, a defective perspiratory mechanism and burn injuries. Heredity is also a well-recognized causative factor.

Healing Options

Home Remedies	- Bakuchi
- Neem
- Manjistha
- Haridra
- Turmeric
Ayurvedic Supplements	- Neem Guard
- Raktasodhak Bati
- Somraji Oil
Diet	- Measures should be adopted to cleanse the system of accumulated toxins. To begin with, the patient should be on juice fast for about a week. After the juice fast, the patient may adopt a restricted diet consisting of fresh fruits, raw or boiled vegetables and whole-meal bread and chapattis. Curd and milk may be added to this diet after a few days. The patient may thereafter gradually embark upon a well-balanced diet of seeds, nuts, grains, vegetables, oil, honey and yeast. The juice fast may be repeated at intervals of two months or so.
- The patient should avoid tea, coffee, alcoholic beverages, all condiments and highly flavoured dishes, sugar, white-flour products, denatured cereals like polished rice and pearl barley and tinned or bottled food.

Lifestyle	• During the initial one-week juice fast, the bowel should be cleansed daily with a lukewarm water enema.
Yoga	• Pranayam • Shirshasan • Pawanmuktasan • Bhujangasan • Sarvangasan

Low Blood Pressure

Low blood pressure or hypotension refers to a fall in blood pressure below normal. It is a condition in which the movement of the heart that pushes blood through the arteries is weak. This may be a direct outcome of a devitalized system.

While the normal limits of blood pressure are defined by the World Health Organization (WHO) as 140mm/Hg systolic and 90 mm/Hg diastolic, it has been now reduced to 120 mm/Hg systolic and 80 mm/Hg diastolic in the United States. Anything above this is considered high blood pressure or hypertension. Anything below this is low blood pressure.

Symptoms

The patient with chronic low blood pressure may complain of lethargy, weakness, fatigue and dizziness. The patient may faint, especially if the arterial pressure continues to drop while standing. These symptoms are presumably due to a decrease in the perfusion of blood to the brain, heart, skeletal muscle and other organs.

Root Causes

The major cause of low blood pressure is poor nutrition. It makes the tissues forming the walls of the blood vessels relaxed, flabby or stretched. This results in less supply of oxygen and nutrients to the tissues. Malnutrition can result from a diet deficient in calories, proteins, vitamin C or almost any one of the B vitamins.

Sometimes blood pressure falls rapidly because of blood loss. Low blood pressure may also develop gradually because of slow bleeding in the gastrointestinal tract, kidneys or bladder. Emotional stress is a far more frequent cause of low blood pressure. To a lesser degree, prolonged disappointments and frustration may result in subnormal blood pressure.

Healing Options

Herbal Home Remedies	• Beetroot • Indian spikenard • Salt • Epsom salt bath
Ayurvedic Supplements	• Stress Guard • Musli Capsules • Ashwagandha Churna • Ashwagandharishta
Diet	• The treatment for low blood pressure should aim at rejuvenation of the whole system. To begin with, the patient should adopt a well-balanced diet with plenty of fresh fruits and vegetables. • Add milk, meat, fish and eggs in the diet. • Opt for grains and vegetables with plenty of salads.
Yoga	• Pranayam (Breathing exercises) • Sarvangasan (Shoulder stand) • Shavasan (Corpse pose) • Padahastasan • Viparita Karani • Trikonasan

Liver Disorder

The most common of all liver ailments, this results in an increase in bile pigments and bilirubin in the blood, giving the skin and mucuos membrane a yellow tinge. It is called *kamala* in Ayurveda.

Symptoms

- Extreme weakness
- Severe headaches
- Constipation
- Nausea
- Yellow discoloration of the eyes, tongue, skin and urine
- Dull ache in the liver region of the stomach
- Possible itching all over the body

Root Causes

- Excessive circulation of pitta (bile pigments) in the blood occurs due to obstruction or impairment of the bile duct, which affects the functioning of the liver or the destruction of the RBCs
- Diseases such as typhoid, malaria, yellow fever and tuberculosis
- Viral infections

Healing Options

Herbal Remedies	- Bhumiamla (*Phyllanthus niruri*) - Ghritkumari (Aloe vera) - Kakmachi (*Solanum nigrum*)
Ayurvedic Supplements	- Livgood Capsule - Livgood Juice - Liverol Syrup - Punarnava Mandoor - Bhumiamla Capsule - Kumariasava
Diet	- Go for a boiled and less spicy diet. - **Vegetables:** Radish leaves, tomato and lemon - **Dry fruits:** Dried dates with almonds and cardamom - Have plenty of sugarcane and orange juice, bitter luffa and barley water. This enhances urination, which helps to eliminate excess bile pigments in the blood.
Yoga	- Sarvangasan - Vajrasan - Ardha Kurmasan - Savasan

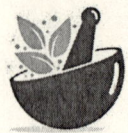

60

Male Sterility

The condition in which a couple has difficulty producing offspring is called sterility. The problem may be either with the male partner or with the female partner. These defects can be either organic or functional. In males, the procreative factor is the sperm. It is produced in the testicles and ejaculated through the male genital organ during sexual intercourse.

The production of sperm is regulated by hormones secreted by the ductless glands of the body. For procreation, the sperm should be active and in sufficient numbers in the semen. Sometimes, because of morbidity, sperm is either less or absent in the semen. In such cases, conception does not occur.

Treatment

The condition in which the sperm does not exist in the semen is difficult to treat. If the sperm are present but they are either few in number or inactive, the condition can be easily remedied.

The root of ashwagandha is the ideal drug for the treatment of this condition. It is cultivated in some parts of the country as jungle weed.

The dried root of this plant can be either taken as a powder in a dose of one teaspoonful twice daily followed by a cup of milk, or it can be boiled with milk. To make it palatable, it can be mixed with sugar syrup. This preparation is called ashwagandha ichya. This linctus (thick liquid medicine) can be given to the patient in a dose of one teaspoonful twice daily, followed by a cup of milk. The alcoholic preparation of this medicine is called ashwagandharishta. It is given to the patient in a dose of 30 ml twice daily after food with an equal quantity of water.

The aforementioned medicines, apart from their spermatogenetic properties, are very good tonics for the nerves and the heart. They do not cause any adverse effects even if used for a long time. They, however, produce warmth in the body. Thus, they are ideal for the winter season.

Healing Options

Ayurvedic Supplements	<ul><li>Vigor 100 Stamina</li><li>Vita-ex Gold</li><li>Musli pak</li><li>Shilajit capsules</li><li>Ashwagandha capsules</li></ul>
Diet	<ul><li>Saline, sour, pungent and bitter things should not be taken in this condition.</li><li>Food ingredients with sweet and astringent taste are normally administered to the patients.</li><li>Milk, ghee and butter are helpful.</li><li>Meat or eggs can be given to patients in good quantity.</li><li>Cow's milk and ghee are considered to be especially useful in this treatment.</li></ul>
Lifestyle	All medicines that produce active sperms of better quality are usually aphrodisiacs, that is, they increase sex drive. The individual should, however, take care not to indulge in sex too frequently. Restraint from sex is always good in this condition.
Yoga	<ul><li>Prayanam</li><li>Padmasan</li><li>Yogamudra</li><li>Garurasan</li><li>Dhanurasan</li><li>Sarvangasan</li></ul>

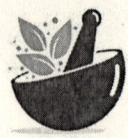

Miscarriage and Abortion

Miscarriage is a term used for the expulsion of the foetus before the term. This occurs mainly during the first trimester of pregnancy, particularly in the third month. However, it can happen at any stage of pregnancy. Miscarriage occurs in two ways—threatened and habitual.

Symptoms

- Pain in the back
- Pallor of face, dull eyes, livid and blotted eyelids
- Feeling of pressure on the pubis, anus and vulva, flabby breast
- Bloody and ichorous discharge from the vagina
- Increased uterine contractions or pain
- Progressive dilation of the cervix

Root Causes

- Insufficient expansion and lack of flexibility of the uterus.
- Accident followed by pain in the back.
- Outer growth (cysts, tumours and carcinomas) of the uterus
- Sexually transmitted diseases

Healing Options

Home Remedies	**For preventing abortion:** • Aparajita • Shatavari • Bidarikand • Barahikand **For preventing excessive bleeding:** • Durba Ras • Kesar (Saffron) • Hirabol • Vasak, haldi and fitkari
Ayurvedic Supplements	• Garbhpal Ras • Garbhchintamani • Lauh Bhasm
Lifestyle	Take as much bed rest as possible.
Yoga	• Viparit Karani with Ashwani Mudra • Supta Bhadrasan with Ashwini Mudra • Utthita Padasan

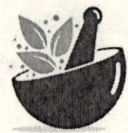

62
Menorrhagia

Excessive bleeding during menstruation is called menorrhagia. In Ayurveda it is known as *rakta pradara*.

Due to hormonal imbalance, excessive bleeding occurs during menstruation. This is caused by the aggravation of pitta. There are other conditions such as uterine cancer and many other diseases in which menorrhagia occurs. Menstruation may start with pain in the abdomen, lumbar region or hips. If the excessive bleeding continues for a longer period, the patient will feel exceedingly debilitating weakness, headache, pain in the calf and restlessness. The patient can turn anaemic and may experience heart palpitations. This may also be associated with breathlessness.

Treatment

Ashoka and lodhra are popularly used for the treatment of this condition. The powder of their barks is given to patients either separately or in a compound form in a dose of one teaspoonful four times a day, with cold water. Ashokarishta and Lodhrasava are two important preparations of these drugs. They are given to the patient in a dose of 30 ml twice daily after food with an equal quantity of water.

The tender leaves of the pomegranate tree are also used for the treatment of this condition. Seven leaves along with seven grains of rice are made into a paste and given to the patient twice daily for a month. This works both as a preventive as well as a curative medicine.

Pravala and mukta are used in acute attacks of this disease. These are also given in powder form called *pishti*. The patient is given 100 g of the powder of this drug four times a day.

Healing Options

Herbal Remedies	• Ashoka • Lodhra
Ayurvedic Supplements	• Meno Guard • Sundarisakhi • Ashokarishta • Lodhrasava
Diet	• Old rice, wheat, moong dal, milk and ghee can be given to the patient. • Sugarcane juice, grapes, jackfruit, banana, amalaki and pomegranate are very useful in this condition. • Hot and spicy food should be strictly avoided.
Lifestyle	• The patient should not resort to any heavy or light exercise. She should take complete rest. Stress, anxiety and anger aggravate this condition. Therefore, complete mental and physical rest is recommended. Exposure to the sun, heat, travelling and long journeys should be avoided. While sleeping, the foot of the bed should be raised a little.
Yoga	• Sarvangasan • Halasan • Bhujangasan • Halasan • Supta Bhadrasan with Ashwini

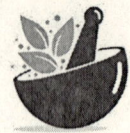

Myopia

Myopia generally occurs in people who have difficulty seeing objects at a distance. This is because of the parallel rays transmitted by the objects focusing in front of the retina. This may be due to a change in the curvature of the refracting surface of the eye or due to abnormal refractivity of the ocular media.

Normally, after the use of spectacles with concave lenses of appropriate curvature, the patient is relieved of the trouble. In one type of myopia, the morbidity continues to increase in adult life. This is called progressive myopia and the patient goes on changing lenses for higher prescription. In Ayurveda this condition is called *drishti dosha*.

In Ayurveda, the person suffering from a chronic cold and constipation is considered more vulnerable to myopia. Nervous debility is also a possible factor.

Symptoms

- Blurred vision
- Watery eyes
- Itching and a feeling of heaviness in the eyeballs
- Burning sensation in the eyes

Root Causes

- Nervous debility
- Chronic cold
- Constipation

Healing Options

Herbs	• Punarnava (for local application) • Jyotishmati • Mamira Ka Surma (for local application) • Triphala
Ayurvedic Supplements	• Saptamrita lauha • Mahatriphala ghrita
Diet	• Pungent and sour food like spices, pickles and curd are contraindicated. • Food that causes constipation and nasal congestion should be avoided. • Fried food should be avoided. • Cow's ghee is considered very useful.
Lifestyle	• The patient should not strain the eyes while studying. • Try to avoid needlework and painting. • The patient is prohibited from staying awake at night, especially to study or watch films.
Yoga	• Pranayam • Padmasan • Meditation • Tadasan • Halasan

64

Memory Loss

Memory helps us to remember what we have previously learnt. For example, when a person remembers a name, they demonstrate that they learnt the name in the past and retained it in the intervening time. While retention is passive, remembering is active and both are part of memory.

Ayurveda considers both body and mind interlinked. No phenomenon is exclusively physical or mental. The body or the mind might predominate in one case and work as a secondary factor in another. Thus, for the treatment of memory loss, both psychological and physical factors are effective.

Treatment

When the power of learning and remembering is impaired, to correct it, a plant called brahmi is popularly used. It is of two types—matsyakshi and mandukparni. These herbs are equally useful in improving memory.

They grow in marshy land near perennial streams. The juice of these plants is used in medicine. About 30 ml of the juice is given to the patient twice daily on an empty stomach. Both are bitter and astringent. They are, therefore, administered with some honey to make them palatable.

Fats are known for their tonic effect on both the heart and brain. Therefore, medicated ghee is made by boiling brahmi, along with other drugs, in pure cow's ghee. This preparation is called brahmighrita. One teaspoonful of this ghee is added to a cup of warm milk, mixed with sugar, and stirred well until it melts and is mixed with the milk. This preparation is more useful when the patient suffering from memory loss is emaciated.

The other drug used by Ayurvedic physicians in the treatment of this condition is called vacha. This also grows in marshy land. The rhizome, or root, of this plant is used in medicines. It is cleaned properly and then ground to a fine powder. One teaspoon of this powder should be given to the patient twice daily, mixed with honey or cow's ghee. Many Ayurvedic preparations for the promotion of memory, like sarasvata churna, contain brahmi and vacha.

Healing Options

Home Remedies	<ul><li>Brahmi</li><li>Jatamanshi</li><li>Sankhapuspi</li><li>Ashwagandha</li></ul>
Ayurvedic Supplements	<ul><li>Stress Guard</li><li>Memorex Tab</li><li>Brahmi Bati</li><li>Sankhapuspi Syrup</li></ul>
Diet	<ul><li>Food ingredients that are sweet and unctuous are useful in this condition.</li><li>Cow's milk, cow's ghee, and other preparations of cow's milk are advisable.</li><li>Pungent and spicy food and bitter and astringent taste should be avoided.</li><li>Almond and almond oil are useful in promoting memory.</li><li>Amlaki can be given to the patient in the form of pickles and vegetables.</li></ul>

| Yoga | - Yogamudra
- Meditation
- Pranayam
- Sarvangasan
- Padahastasan
- Sasangasan |

Note

All the aforementioned medicines act well when one is at peace mentally. Therefore, care should be taken to keep the patient free from stress, anxiety and strain. They should be advised to follow religious practices and religious prayers. Meditation according to the method prescribed in yoga serves a very useful purpose in promoting and correcting memory.

Migraine (Severe Headache with Nausea)

Migraine is a paroxysmal ailment, accompanied by severe headache, generally on one side of the head, and associated with disorders of the digestion, liver and vision. It usually occurs when a person is under great mental stress or has suddenly gotten over that state.

Migraine usually occurs suddenly. The head and neck muscles become overworked due to continuous stress. The tightened muscles squeeze the arteries and reduce blood flow. Thus, when the person relaxes, suddenly the constricted muscles expand, stretching the walls of the blood vessels. With each heartbeat, the blood pushes through these vessels and expands them further, causing intense pain.

Symptoms

There is a definite pattern of migraine. The pain is experienced on only one side of the head and often radiates from the eye. The right side of the head may be affected in one attack, and the next time, the concentration of pain may be on the left side.

Migraine attacks are usually preceded by short periods of depression, irritability and loss of appetite. Some people get daily attacks, others every month or every two to three months. The main symptoms of migraine are pounding pain, nausea and vomiting. The blood vessels on the affected side of the head become prominent and pulsating.

A migraine gives a fair warning before striking. The patient sees flashes of light or black spots or only parts of the objects in front of them. They may also feel numbness or weakness in an arm or leg or on one side of the face.

Root Causes

A migraine may also result from a variety of causes like low blood sugar, allergy, infection, excessive intake of some drugs, weak constitution, low energy, nutritional deficiency, overwork, improper sleep and rest, excessive smoking and drinking. Menstruation in women is also an important cause of migraine. This form of migraine usually abates after menopause.

Healing Options

Home Remedies	• Grapes • Vegetable juices • Carrot with spinach • Carrot with beet
Ayurvedic Supplements	• Shadbindu Taila • Stress Guard • Baidyanath Balm • Sirasuladi Vajra Ras
Diet	• At first, the patient should take a liquid diet like fruit juices, vegetable juices, milk, soup, etc. After that, they can embark upon a light diet like boiled vegetables, fruits, grains, or any lightly cooked food. Gradually, they may start a normal diet.

Lifestyle	• During the initial one or two days, only liquids like milk and juice should be taken. • Keep the bowels clean. • Try to avoid stress and anxiety. • Spend time with your children and pets. • Walking in the morning and evening helps to overcome these complications.
Yoga	• Pranayam • Padmasan • Meditation • Ardha Kurmasan • Sahaj Ustrasan

66

Measles

Measles is an acute, infectious disease that occurs mostly in children. The tender the age, the better the ability to fight off the disease. This infectious disease is characterized by the catarrh of the respiratory passages and a widespread eruption on the skin. In Ayurveda this is known as *romantika*.

Symptoms and Causes

According to Ayurveda, measles is a result of vitiation of both kapha and pitta.

Measles is caused by a type of virus called paramyxovirus. It is an extremely contagious infection that spreads through the tiny droplets present in the air when an individual carrying the virus sneezes or coughs.

Measles usually occurs during the spring and autumn seasons. In the beginning, the patient gets cough, cold and fever. The eyes turn red, followed by drowsiness, anorexia and even diarrhoea. Eruptions start from the forehead, and they are small and red. In about three to four days, this spreads all over the body. When the eruptions fully disappear, the fever subsides, and other accompanying symptoms like cough and cold also go away.

Healing Options

Home Remedies	• At first, have the patient wear warm clothes. • Hot water and other liquids should be given to avoid dehydration. • A powder of equal parts of tamarind seeds and turmeric may be given thrice daily.
Ayurvedic Supplements	• Neem Guard • Prawal Pishti • Swarnamakshika Bhasma
Diet	• The patient should be given a very light diet like barley gruel and fruit juice.
Lifestyle	• Patients should not be exposed to draughts; they are advised to lie down in a soft bed in a slightly darkened room. Bathing during the attack of the disease is strictly prohibited.
Yoga	• Bhujangasan (Prevention purpose only) • Pawanmuktasan (Prevention purpose only) • Sarvangasan (Prevention purpose only)

67
Obesity

What is Obesity?

In Ayurveda this condition is called *medoroga*. Obesity is caused by the accumulation of excessive fat in the body. It can cause serious health conditions affecting the functions of vital organs like the heart, liver and kidneys. It might also give way to diabetes.

Root Causes

- Intake of excessive calories
- Complete lack of mental and physical exercise
- In rare cases, disturbances of thyroid or pituitary glands
- Excessive and regular consumption of alcohol

Symptoms

- Abnormal girth and extra weight, which hinders normal life activity
- Increases chances of getting heart diseases and diabetes
- Breathlessness, even on the slightest exertion
- Development of asthmatic tendencies

Healing Options

Home Remedies	• Guggulu (*Commiphora mukul*) • Punarnava (*Boerhaavia diffusa*)

Ayurvedic Supplements	• Ezi Slim Plus • Ezi Slim Juice • Medohar Vidangadi Lauh • Punarnavadi Guggul
Diet	• Avoid carbohydrates and high-fat food. • Thrive on plenty of water and juices like lemon, grapefruit, orange and pineapple. • Add garden-fresh salads, raw green vegetables and fresh fruits to your low-calorie diet.
Lifestyle	• Exercise religiously through activities like walking, swimming and cycling. • Think positive. • Take sauna and steam baths and regular massages. • Opt for Panchakarma.
Yoga	• Pranayam • Salbhasan • Trikonasan • Pawanmuktasan • Utthita Padmasan

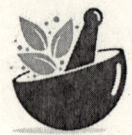

68

Oedema

Oedema is the condition of accumulation of excess water in the tissues.

Symptoms

Non-inflammatory swelling of various parts of the body

Root Causes

Ailments of the heart, liver, kidney and anaemia

Healing Options

Home Remedies	• Punarnava (*Borhaavia diffusa*) • Hasti Sundi (*Heliotropium indicum*)
Ayurvedic Supplements	• Sothari Mandur • Sothari Lauh • Punarnavaristha
Diet	• Strictly avoid fried and fatty food, salt and curd. • Go for vegetables like drumsticks, green bananas, gourd, patola, bitter gourd and ripe papaya.
Lifestyle	• Do not indulge in daytime naps. • Move more and avoid sedentary habits.

Yoga	• Right-nostril pranayam • Meditation • Viparit karani • Halasan • Sarvangasan
Ayurvedic Massage	Ayurvedic massage with Punarnawadi Tel

69

Perimenopause

Menopause is a natural phase of a woman's life, not a disease or a health crisis. However, menopause may occur when many other changes are happening in a person's life. For instance, children may be getting married or leaving home, parents may be ill or dying, or one may be wondering what they will do after retiring from work. So, it is important to manage it in one's daily life, and understand what to expect and also the possible effects.

Menopause marks the stage when women stop ovulating. It happens when the ovaries stop releasing the ovum, usually a gradual process. Sometimes, it happens all at once.

Menopause affects each woman differently. Some start early, some start and stop, but most experience the change around the age of fifty. It usually lasts up to five years. While oestrogen levels drop during the post-menopausal period, the hormones do not completely disappear.

Symptoms like hot flashes, dizziness, headache, difficulty breathing, shortness of breath, heart palpitations and depression may be caused by oestrogen deficiency. If one is hypoglycaemic, the symptoms are often more pronounced. Stress puts a burden on the adrenal glands, causing them to overwork. Therefore, these glands produce fewer amounts of the hormones that are needed to reduce the side effects of the menopause. Hot flashes usually occur because of blood vessel dilation.

What is perimenopause?

Perimenopause is the period of gradual changes that lead to menopause. It affects a woman's hormones, body and emotions. It can be a stop-start process that may take months or years. 'Climacteric' is another word for the time when a woman passes from the reproductive to the non-reproductive years of her life.

The production of oestrogen by ovaries slows down during perimenopause. Hormone levels fluctuate, causing changes just as they did during adolescence. The changes leading to menopause may seem more intense than those during puberty.

An induced menopause occurs when the ovaries are removed or damaged as in hysterectomy or chemotherapy. In this case, menopause begins immediately, with no perimenopause. The time after menopause is called post-menopause.

There is a growing interest in the natural approach to minimizing the effects of menopause. Many women are concerned about the side effects of conventional medicine and find herbal solutions remarkably effective. This is practised in traditional Chinese medicine, which has been around for thousands of years.

Herbal formulations are designed to increase the body's ability to produce its own oestrogen and revitalize body functions. Additionally, some books are effective in assisting women through this difficult time.

Causes

During a woman's reproductive years, the monthly release of eggs from the ovaries provides a continuous flow of progesterone and oestrogen, hormones necessary for a successful pregnancy.

With age, a woman's body no longer releases the signals that induce the ovulation of eggs from the ovaries. The result is a measurable decrease in the associated hormones and normal menstruation. This also reduces the body's ability to maintain calcium levels and leads to the loss of minerals from the bones. The net loss of calcium is a combination of changes in calcium excretion and calcium absorption.

Symptoms

As most women approach menopause, their menstrual periods become irregular. This happens either closer together or further apart.

Other common symptoms include:

- Achy joints
- Decrease or changes in sexual desire or in the ability to concentrate or recall
- Extreme sweating
- Headaches
- Frequent urination
- Early awakening
- Vaginal dryness
- Mood changes
- Insomnia
- Night sweats
- Conditions commonly associated with premenstrual syndrome (PMS)

A woman may have some or none of these symptoms. The symptoms can be very unpredictable and disturbing if a woman is unaware they are related to menopause.

A woman's experiences during menopause may also be influenced by the following life changes:

- Changes in domestic, social and personal relationships
- Changes in identity and body image
- Divorce or widowhood

- Retirement
- Increased anxiety about illness, ageing and death
- Loss of friends, loved ones and financial security
- Anxiety about the loss of independence, disability or loneliness

An increasing number of women going through perimenopause also have young children to care for.

Whatever the cause or circumstance, the conditions women experience before and after menopause are very real and sometimes need medical attention. All women face an increased risk of heart disease and osteoporosis after menopause.

Healing Options

Ayurvedic Supplements	<ul><li>Zest Female</li><li>Stress Guard</li><li>Sundari Kalp</li><li>Sundari Kalp Forte</li></ul>
Lifestyle	<ul><li>As mentioned earlier, menopause may occur when many other changes are happening in you. This is why it is probably more helpful to think of how your daily activities and lifestyle will affect menopause. For instance, exercising and eating right can make a real difference in how you feel and even help prevent some of the long-term effects that are linked to oestrogen deficiency (like heart disease or osteoporosis).</li><li>Physical changes do occur with menopause and ageing. However, the changes that happen during this period can be minimized by healthy living and developing a sense of purpose in life.</li></ul>

| Yoga | • Pranayam
• Sarvangasan
• Vrikshasan
• Trikonasan |

70

Piles

Called *arsha* in Ayurveda and categorized as dry and bleeding, it is the condition of the presence of varicose veins in the anal region.

Symptoms

- Intense pain at the time of passing stool
- Profuse bleeding leading to anaemia
- Itching in the rectal region
- Wind formation in the stomach
- Sitting becomes problematic

Root Causes

- Chronic constipation and other bowel disorders
- The pressure exerted to evacuate the constipated bowels affects the surrounding veins causing piles.
- Prolonged periods of sitting or standing
- Strenuous work
- Obesity
- Mental stress
- Hereditary factors
- Pregnancy

Healing Options

Home Remedies	• Haritaki (*Terminalia chebula*) • Jimikand (*Amorphophallus campanulatus*)
Ayurvedic Supplements	• Piloss capsules • Pirrhoids tablets • Pirrhoids ointment • Arshoghani Bati • Abhyaristha
Diet	• Avoid potatoes, yellow variety of pumpkin and colocasia. • Go for the following diet: **Seeds:** Mango seeds, sesame seeds **Fresh fruits:** Jambul, dry figs, papaya, amalaki **Vegetables:** Radish, turnip, bitter gourd, onion and ginger **Grains:** Rice, wheat
Lifestyle	• Exercise is a must. • Avoid horse rides or sitting on hard seats. • Drink lots of water.
Yoga	• Bhujangasan (Cobra pose) • Dhanurasan (Bow pose) • Viparit karani • Pawanmuktasan • Utthitha Padmasan
Ayurvedic Massage	• Kasisadi Taila

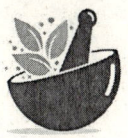

Premenstrual Syndrome (PMS)

From puberty to entire adulthood of any woman, oestrogen and progesterone are the main hormones that play a key role in her life. These ensure the menstrual cycle is regular and comes to a natural halt only during pregnancy and after a certain age. However, before the onset of menstruation every month, some women often experience psychological and physiological changes.

Symptoms

- Depression
- Headaches
- Backache
- Fullness of the breasts
- Swelling in the lower extremities
- Insomnia

Root Causes

- Hormonal changes
- Anxiety

Healing Options

| Home Remedies | • Chitrak mool (*Plumbago zeylanica*)
• Nirgundi (*Vitex negundo*) |

Ayurvedic Supplements	• Stress Guard • Sundari Sakhi • Rajahpravartini Bati • Kumaryasava
Diet	• Have plenty of water, fruit juices and soups. • Go for a nutritive diet, complete with cereals, green salads, boiled vegetables and milk. • Avoid white-flour products, rich cakes, pastries, spicy food, pickles, strong tea and coffee.
Lifestyle	• Try to keep your bowels regular. • Go for a cold tub bath. • Avoid smoking and consumption of alcohol.
Ayurvedic Massage	• Massage the chest and the back twice a day for 20 minutes with Mahanarayan Tel.
Yoga	• Bhujangasan (Cobra pose) • Halasan (Plough pose) • Bhadrasan • Baddhakonasan • Supta Bhadrasan

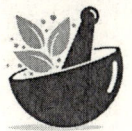

72

Pyorrhoea

Pyorrhoea, or periodontal disease, to give it a proper medical term, is a disease of the gums. It is one of the most widely prevalent diseases. It affects the membrane surrounding the roots of the teeth and leads to loosening of the teeth, pus formation and shrinkage of gums. This disease is the primary cause of tooth loss among adults.

Symptoms

The gums become tender, and on pressing, pus oozes out along the margin of the teeth. The pus from the cavities continually finds its way into the stomach. When the disease is far advanced, the gums become swollen, and the stomach, soused with increasing quantities of pus, does not function properly. Sepsis may appear in various forms; digestion gets disturbed, liver issues set in, and the whole system is adversely affected.

Root Causes

Pyorrhoea is triggered by bacterial activity. A thin layer of harmful bacteria continuously builds up on our teeth. If it is not removed by tooth cleansing, especially after meals, it forms an organized mass on the tooth surface in a short time. This is referred to as bacterial plaque.

The bacteria in plaque produce many toxins, which irritate the gums, causing them to become inflamed, tender, and prone to bleeding easily. The bacterial activity is, however, facilitated by the lowered vitality of the system. Other factors contributing to the development of pyorrhoea include chemical irritants in the mouth, improper brushing, stagnation of food particles and improper use of toothpicks.

Healing Options

Home Remedies	• Guava leaves • Lemon and lime • Spinach juice • Wheat
Ayurvedic Applications	• Dant Manjan Lal (powder) • Lavang Tel • Irimedadi Taila
Diet	• The patient should take only boiled vegetables, fruit juices and fruits first. • Oranges and carrots should be taken at first. After the juice fast, the patient can take three normal meals per day, but he or she must take properly cooked food. • White bread, white sugar and tinned food must be avoided. • Condiments, sauces, alcohol, coffee and strong tea as well as meat and other fleshy food should be avoided.
Lifestyle	• During the juice fast, the bowels should be cleaned daily with a warm water enema. • Daily dry friction and hip bath as well as breathing and other exercises should form a part of the morning routine. • A hot Epsom salt bath taken twice weekly will also be beneficial.

| Yoga | • Trikonasan
• Viparita Karani
• Sarvangasan |

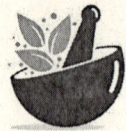

73

Psoriasis
(Scaly Disorder of the Skin)

Psoriasis is one of the most stubborn skin diseases. It is a chronic disease characterized by thick, red, silvery and scaly patches on the skin. This disease affects both sexes equally and is more common during the first 15 to 30 years, although it may appear at any age. Psoriasis is not contagious.

Symptoms

The skin of the person suffering from psoriasis is irritated and may be covered with bright silvery scales. Sometimes there is also itching. The areas usually involved are the elbows, knees, the skin behind the ears and the scalp. The disease may also affect the underarms and the genital area. The lesions vary in size from minute papules to sheets covering large parts of the body. Quite often, the discs measure half an inch to several inches. The lesions are always dry and rarely infected.

Root Causes

Recent studies have shown that psoriasis involves an abnormality in the mechanism by which the skin grows and replaces itself. The abnormality is related to the metabolism of amino acids—nature's basic building blocks for the reproduction of cell tissues. Heredity also plays a role in the development of psoriasis, as it tends to occur in families. The factors that aggravate and precipitate the outbreak of these diseases are physical and emotional stress, infections, and the use of certain medicines for the treatment of other diseases.

Healing Options

Home Remedies	• Avocado oil • Cashew nut oil • Buttermilk • Vitamin E
Ayurvedic Supplements/ Applications	• Neem Guard • Liverol Strong • Neem oil • Chalmugra oil (Tubrak)
Diet	• Psoriasis is a metabolic disease. It is essential to eat less spicy and easily digestible food. • Fruits, vegetables and fruit juices are very helpful. • Bitter gourd, curd, boiled vegetables and pumpkin are recommended. • Animal fats, eggs and processed canned food should be avoided.
Lifestyle	• Keep the bowels clean. • Keep your towel and clothes separate and clean. • Try taking a bath with an Ayurvedic soap that contains neem. • If possible, try a seawater bath or apply seawater to the affected place once a day. • Keep your skin clean.
Yoga	• Padahastasan • Pawanmuktasan • Bhujangasan

Peptic Ulcer (Stomach Ulcer)

A peptic ulcer refers to a lesion in the inner lining of the stomach and the adjoining intestinal tract called the duodenum. The ulcer located in the stomach is known as a gastric ulcer, and that located in the duodenum is called a duodenal ulcer. Usually, both are grouped and termed peptic ulcer. In Ayurveda it is a disease of the tri-doshic nature. However, an aggravation of pitta is noted in all cases.

Symptoms

A peptic ulcer is the result of hyperacidity, which is caused by an increase in hydrochloric acid in the stomach. This strong acid, secreted by the cells lining the stomach, erodes the inner lining of the stomach.

Dietetic indiscretions such as overeating, taking heavy meals or highly-spiced food, coffee, alcohol and smoking are the main factors contributing to this condition. Other causes are the ingestion of certain drugs, food poisoning, certain infections, gout, emotional disturbances, stress and nervous tension.

Causes

The symptoms of peptic ulcer include severe pain and discomfort in the upper part of the abdomen. Gastric ulcer pain usually occurs an hour after meals and rarely at night. Duodenal ulcer pain usually occurs between meals when the stomach is empty.

The pain is relieved by food, especially milk. As the disease progresses, there is distension of the stomach due to excessive flatulence, mental stress, insomnia and a gradual weakening of the body. Blood may be detected in the stool.

Healing Options

Herbal Home Remedies	<ul><li>Banana</li><li>Bansalochan</li><li>Chandan</li><li>Lime</li><li>Vegetable juice</li><li>Almond milk</li></ul>
Ayurvedic Supplements	<ul><li>Acidity Guard</li><li>Diagest Guard Juice</li><li>Ayucid</li><li>Avipattikar Churna</li><li>Mahashankha Bati</li><li>Prawal Bhasma</li></ul>
Diet	<ul><li>The diet of the patient suffering from peptic ulcer should be planned to provide adequate nutrition, while affording rest to the disturbed organs, maintaining continuous neutralization of the gastric acid, inhibiting the production of acid and reducing mechanical and chemical irritation.</li><li>Milk, cream, butter, fruits, fresh raw and boiled vegetables, natural food, and natural vitamin supplements constitute the best diet.</li></ul>
Lifestyle	<ul><li>Daily massages and deep breathing exercises are helpful. Above all, the patient must try to rid himself of worries and stay cheerful. They should also cultivate regularity in their habits—be it work, exercise or rest.</li></ul>

Yoga	<ul><li>Vajrasan</li><li>Padmasan</li><li>Pawanmuktasan</li><li>Bhujangasan</li><li>Paschimothanasan</li><li>Siddhayoni Asan</li><li>Savasan</li></ul>

Prostate Disorder

A large percentage of men over 50 years of age suffer from prostate issues of one form or another. The prostate gland is a male gland, comparable in shape and size to a large chestnut. It is situated at the base of the urinary bladder and around the beginning of the urethra. There are various types of prostate disorders, the more important being hypertrophy or enlargement of the prostate gland, and prostatitis or inflammation of the prostate gland.

Symptoms

There are two warning signals to indicate the possibility of prostate disorders. The first is the interference with the passage of urine, and the second is the need to urinate frequently during the night's sleep. Other symptoms are a dull pain in the lower back and pain in the hips, legs and feet.

Causes

The position of the prostate gland is prone to congestion and other disorders. In a standing position, the pressure falls on the pelvic region just where the prostate gland is situated. With ageing, the body gets heavier and loses its flexibility. This puts greater pressure on the pelvis and increases the vulnerability of the prostate gland. Prolonged sitting in certain occupations also increases the pressure on the pelvic region. Acute prostatitis may also result from exposure to cold and infectious diseases. Another important cause of prostate disorders is constipation.

Healing Options

Herbal Home Remedies	• Pumpkin seeds • Vegetable juices • Zinc (Yasad Bhasma)
Ayurvedic Supplements	• Prosguard • Prostaid • Chandraprabha Bati • Shilajit tablets or capsules • Gokshuradi Guggulu
Diet	• To begin with, the patient should avoid all solid food and subsist on water mixed with a little lemon juice for two or three days. The water may be drunk cold or hot and should be taken every hour or so during waking hours. This increases urine formation. • After fasting for a few days, the patient may adopt an all-fruit diet, consisting of juicy fruits, for the next three days. This should be followed by a diet consisting of two meals of fruits and one of cooked vegetables for seven days. • Thereafter, the patient may adopt a well-balanced diet, with emphasis on seeds, nuts, grains, vegetables and fruits. • Heavy starches, sweet stimulants, and highly seasoned food should be entirely avoided, as they are said to cause direct irritation to the prostate gland and bladder.

Lifestyle	• During the initial water fast of two to three days, an enema may be taken once a day to clear the bowel of accumulations. • Hot and cold applications are highly beneficial in the treatment of prostate disorders. • After a thorough cleansing through a warm water enema, hot and cold applications may be used directly on the prostate gland. • Irregularities in eating and drinking habits, long periods of sitting, and vigorous exercise should be avoided. All efforts should be made to tone up the general condition of the body.
Yoga	• Vajrasan • Paschimottanasan

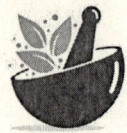

Palpitations

Palpitation, a common problem, is a state in which the heart beats violently and irregularly. It is a distressing condition, but it is not always serious.

Symptoms

The main symptom of palpitation of the heart is a kind of 'thumping' feeling in the chest. The patient feels discomfort in the chest. The pulse may become faster than normal.

Causes

Heart palpitations may occur due to a variety of factors, most of which may not be related to the heart. Anything that increases the workload of the heart may bring up this condition. Some people may experience palpitations while lying on the left side because the heart is closer to the chest wall in this position. Usually, nervous people suffer from this condition. Although palpitations occur as other symptoms in serious heart diseases, the majority of the cases are due to anxiety and have no direct connection with heart disease. Other causes contributing to this condition are an overfull stomach, flatulence and constipation. Excessive smoking may also give rise to this disorder.

Healing Options

Herbal Home Remedies	• Grapes • Ashwagandha • Satabari • Brahmi
Ayurvedic Supplements	• Stress Guard • Keshari Kalp • Ashwagandharishta • Brahmi Bati
Diet	• The patient experiencing heart palpitations should take a simple diet consisting of natural food, with an emphasis on fresh fruits and raw or lightly cooked vegetables. • They should avoid tea, coffee, alcohol, chocolate, soft drinks, food colourings, white rice and condiments. • They should restrict their diet to three meals a day. • They should eat fruits, milk, a handful of nuts or seeds, and fresh vegetables.
Lifestyle	• The patient should meditate every day. • Swimming, skipping and cycling are good for health.
Yoga	• Pranayam • Sarvangasan • Shavasan • Padmasan • Gomukhasan • Savasan

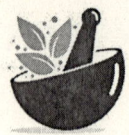

Painful Menstruation

In Ayurveda this disorder is known as *rajah-kriccha*. Ayurveda attributes painful menstruation to the predominance of the doshas. The pain may appear before the menstruation starts and may subside thereafter. It may also continue till the end of menstruation. The pain affects the lower pelvic region and, at times, it becomes severe. The patient might experience nausea, vomiting, loss of appetite, constipation and disturbed sleep.

Treatment

In Ayurveda, the pelvis is considered the seat of *apana vayu*, which is responsible for the elimination of menstrual blood, stools, urine, ovum and sperm (in males). Women prone to constipation are therefore recommended to take a purgative two days before the date of menstruation. Ashoka is the drug of choice for the treatment of this condition. From its pulp, the juice is extracted and given to the patient. Sometimes the juice is dehydrated and the powder obtained is used as medicine. This plant grows in all parts of India and abundantly in deserts and rocky regions.

Ashokarishta, which is an alcoholic preparation of this drug, is given to the patient in a dose of four teaspoons, twice daily after food with an equal quantity of water. Rajapravartini Bati, which contains borax in Bhasma form, asafoetida and kumara, is also an effective drug. Two tablets of these medicines are given to the patient twice a day for about seven days, immediately before the due date of the menses. It relieves congestion in the pelvic organs and works as a laxative, thus keeping the patient free from pain during menstruation.

Pain during menstruation might be caused due to an organic defect in the female genital tract. In this case, surgery is the only option. Medicines prescribed will be helpful only if the pain is caused by functional defects.

Healing Options

Ayurvedic Supplements	• Sundari Sakhi • Rajahparvartini Bati • Ashokarishta
Diet	• The patient should not be given fried food, pulses and sour things. • The last week of the menstrual cycle is very crucial for the patient. They should not take anything that will cause constipation. • Vegetables like colocasia, potato, yellow pumpkin and brinjal are to be avoided. • White pumpkin, papaya, surana, drumstick, bitter gourd and cucumber are useful. Garlic is especially recommended. • Women with painful menstrual cycles should use garlic in a dose of ten cloves, twice a day. The outer coating of garlic should be removed and cut into pieces. The pungent smell of garlic is reduced when a little bit of buttermilk or lime juice is added to it. If, however, the patient is unable to tolerate the residual smell of garlic, it should be fried with a little butter.

	• As has been mentioned earlier, impairment of apana vayu is primarily responsible for this trouble. Its normal course is downwards, and if it does not move, then it is because of hormonal imbalance, constipation, or any other factor. The best thing to do is to add a sufficient quantity of asafoetida to the food of the patient. It can be given to the patient in a powder form and for this, it is fried with ghee or butter in a big spoon over fire. This makes it brittle, and powder can be made from it conveniently. This powder should be taken in hot water. Because of the pungent smell it emits, some people do not like to take it alone. It may be added with buttermilk or vegetables or rice or bread.
Lifestyle	• The patient should walk at least three to four kilometres a day. A morning walk is extremely useful in this condition. • The patient should try to reduce their weight. • Some physical exercises involving the bending of the waist region and contraction of the pelvic muscles should be done regularly. • Sleeping during the daytime is extremely harmful. • During the period of menstruation, the patient should take complete rest.
Yoga	• Surya Namaskar • Pawanmuktasan • Bhujangasan • Bhujangasan • Ek Pada Salavasan • Bhadrasan with Ashwini Mudra

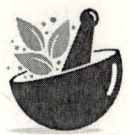

Premature Ejaculation

Lack of ejaculatory control is a very common sexual issue among men. Premature ejaculation occurs when semen leaves a man's body sooner than desired.

However, most people tend to forget that premature ejaculation is relative to the man and his partner's expectations.

One might now ask, 'What is normal or typical?' Let's first, however, consider the question, 'What is natural?' Although averages stated vary a bit from study to study, it is safe to say that the average healthy male under 30 ejaculates in 1 to 3 minutes.

Healing Options

Herbal Remedies	• Asparagus (*Safed Musli*) • Garlic • Drumstick
Ayurvedic Supplements	• Vigor 100 Stamina • Vita-Ex Gold • Musli X • Musli Pak • Shilajit tablets or capsules
Ayurvedic Oils for Massage	• Vita-Ex Massage Oil • Sri Gopal Tel

Diet	- Diet is an important factor; one should adopt an exclusive fresh-fruit diet. Take fresh fruits and fresh fruit juice twice daily. - Food such as nuts, cereals, vegetables, fruits, milk and honey should be taken. - Avoid smoking, alcohol, tea, coffee and all processed, canned, refined and denatured food, especially white sugar and white flour and products made from them.
Lifestyle	- Take medicines (aphrodisiacs or stimulants) that produce active sperms of better quality.
Yoga	- Sarvangasan - Halasan - Matsyasan - Gomukhasan - Baddhakonasan - Supta Bhadrasan with Ashwini Mudra

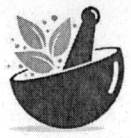

Premature Baldness

Baldness is the loss of hair on the head. It is called *khalitya* in Ayurveda.

Symptoms

Premature baldness may be due to certain serious diseases like acute fever, myxedema (a syndrome caused by hypothyroidism), syphilis, influenza, anaemia, anxiety or nervous shock. If premature baldness is hereditary, not much can be done except delaying the falling of the hair for a few years through proper medication. Sometimes, eczema and psoriasis of the scalp lead to rapid baldness.

Root Causes

The administration of drugs indicates that medication for premature greying of the hair does help in cases of baldness, but recourse to medication must be taken at an earlier stage. If the hair has fallen out and the follicles have closed, nothing much can be done.

Ayurvedic Supplements and Massage Oils	- Arogyavardhini Vati - Mahabhringraj Tel - Bhringrajasava
Diet	- Patients should only take milk and sugar and avoid salt as much as possible. - Sour food like yoghurt is not helpful. - Pungent, hot and spicy food should be avoided.
Lifestyle	- If the baldness is due to any of the aforementioned serious diseases, the medication should start right from the moment the falling of the hair is noticed. - A natural remedy is mahabhringraj oil. It should be massaged into the scalp with the fingers and left on for at least an hour before taking a bath.
Yoga	- Sarvangasan - Viparita Karani (prevention purpose only) - Padahastasan (prevention purpose only)

80

Rheumatism

Characterized by intense pain and inflammation of the muscles, ligaments, tendons and joints, it is termed amavata in Ayurveda. Divided into chronic muscular rheumatism (affecting the muscles) and chronic articular rheumatism (affecting the joints), if neglected, it can even affect the heart.

Symptoms

- Fever
- Immense pain and stiffness in the affected muscles in case of chronic muscular rheumatism
- Excruciating pain and stiffness in the joints in case of chronic articular rheumatism

Root Causes

- Accumulation of toxins in the joints caused by improper digestion, metabolism or excretion.
- Teeth, tonsils and gallbladder infections
- Aggravated by exposure to cold weather

Healing Options

Home Remedies	• Sallai Guggul (*Boswellia sarrata*) • Guggulu (*Commiphora mukul*) • Rasna (*Vanda roxburghii*) • Lohsun (*Allium sativum*)

Ayurvedic Supplements	- Arth Plus - Arth Oil - Rumartho Gold - Yograj Guggul - Rashnadi Guggul - Maharashnadi Kadha
Diet	- Avoid curd and all sour food, pulses (except moong dal), rice, meat, fish, white bread, sugar, refined cereals, fried food, tea or coffee. - Have potato and lemon juice. - Celery seeds and bitter gourd are highly beneficial.
Lifestyle	- Bowels should be cleansed daily. - Soak the affected parts in hot water containing Epsom salt. Then apply Mahabishgarbh oil. - Hot water bag to the affected area is extremely beneficial. - Avoid damp places and exposure to cold weather. - Don't indulge in daytime sleeping. - Limit yourself to restricted exercise.
Yoga	- Halasan - Dhanurasan - Ardha Chandrasan - Tadasan - Bhujangasan
Ayurvedic Massage	- Mahanaryan Taila - Mahamas Taila - Saindhavadi Taila - Rhuma Oil

81

Ringworm

Ringworm is a fungal infection of the scalp or skin. Ringworm on the scalp may leave a flaky patch of baldness. It causes a reddish, ring-shaped rash that may itch or burn. The area may be dry and scaly or moisy and crusty. The same fungi that infect humans can also infect animals such as dogs and cats. Infections may be acquired from pets and infected children.

Ringworm spreads through direct contact with a person or animal infected with the fungus. It can also spread indirectly through contact with objects (combs or clothing) or surfaces that have been contaminated with the fungus. The fungus is no longer present when the lesion starts to shrink.

Root Causes

Ringworm infection can occur on the scalp, body, feet or nails. Ringworm of the scalp is common among children because of the lack of protective fatty acids in their scalp. The disease spreads on the skin and penetrates deeper into the hair roots. The affected hair becomes dull and breaks off near the root. This leaves bald spots on the scalp.

The patches of ringworm on the body are usually round or oval, with raised pink and scaly rings that show a clean space in the centre. The itching on the infected parts of the body if not treated for a long time, becomes chronic and is difficult to get rid of.

Symptoms

Ringworm is passed from an infected person to a healthy person by contact. It can also spread by the use of the towel of an infected person.

Healing Options

Home Remedies	• Neem • Holy basil • Turmeric
Ayurvedic Supplements	• Neem Guard • Neem oil • Mahamarichyadi Taila • Haridrakhand (VRI) • Daad Malham
Diet	• Patients should eat plenty of fresh vegetable juices, fruit juices, fresh salads and fruits. • They should avoid canned or packed food. • They should eat rice, vegetables, fresh fish, dal and roti. • It's recommended that they avoid tea, coffee, alcohol, etc.
Lifestyle	• Patients should get as much fresh air as possible. • They should drink plenty of water and bathe twice daily. • Coconut oil may be applied on the affected part; sunbathing is also beneficial. • Maintain a good handwashing technique among children and adults. • Prohibit sharing of personal items, such as hair-care articles, towels and clothing. • Dry skin thoroughly after washing. • Wash bathroom surfaces daily.
Yoga	• Vajrasan • Halasan • Viparit Karani

82

Sinusitis

Sinusitis refers to an inflammation of the mucous membrane lining the paranasal sinuses. It is often a result of a common cold, influenza, and other general infections. Germs sometimes find their way into these sinuses on either side of the nasal passage leading to health problems. In Ayurveda it means that kapha is vitiated in most cases.

Symptoms

Recurrent common cold is the first stage of this disease, followed by these symptoms:

- Excessive or constant sneezing
- Runny nose
- Blockage of the nostrils
- Pain in the forehead and below the eyes
- Low-grade fever
- Lack of appetite
- Difficulty breathing
- Heaviness in the head

Root Causes

- Increase of kapha in the body
- Infection caused after catching a cold or allergy due to dust, pollen, damp and cold weather

Healing Options

Home Remedies	- Tulsi (*Ocimum santum*) - Kantakari (*Solanum xanthocarpum*) - Vasaka (*Adhatoda vasica*)
Ayurvedic Supplements	- Immune Guard - Allergy Guard - Shadbindu Taila - Godanti Bhasma - Mahalakshmivilas Ras
Diet	- Maintain a diet of low-calorie food, raw fruits and vegetables with plenty of fruit juice. - Eat well-balanced food including seeds, nuts, grains, vegetables and fruits. - Patients should avoid fried and starchy food like white sugar, white flour, macaroni, pies, cakes and candies.
Lifestyle	- Patients should avoid perfumes and strongly scented hair or oil. - Avoid exposure to cold and damp weather.
Yoga	- Matsyasan - Halasan - Dhanurasan - Ardhakurmasan - Sasangasan - Ustrasan

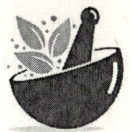

83

Skin Care

Skin and nails provide a look at the inner health of the body. These outward 'signs' can tell you a lot about the condition of your inward health.

Often, we may have problems with our skin, such as dull skin, skin likely to break out in blotches, or skin that dehydrates easily. All these problems and many more indicate a lack of proper nutrition.

Poor diet, drugs, alcohol, excessive sun exposure, environmental toxins and tobacco smoke increase free radical damage and decrease enzyme activity. Both free radical damage and the reduction in enzyme activity can increase the appearance of wrinkles, age spots and sagging skin and ultimately can also lead to skin cancer.

Free radicals oxidize cells, making normal cell metabolism impossible. Enzymes can help prevent or treat skin damage by fighting these free radicals and reducing stress on the body system.

The skin, the largest organ and composed primarily of collagen, reflects our overall health and acts as a barrier against the outside world. Collagen fibres form an elastin network that makes up connective tissues. The skin's elasticity, strength and smoothness come from the makeup of collagen fibres.

Functions of the Skin

- Protects internal organs and tissues from injury
- Preserves valuable moisture and helps maintain normal body temperature
- Protects the body from toxins, viruses and bacteria

Measuring Skin's Vitality
To measure the amount of free radical damage, you must perform the skin elasticity test. Grasp the skin on the back of the hand between the thumb and index finger. Raise the skin and release it. The skin fold should immediately flatten. If a ridge remains, the skin is ageing and damaged by the coalescence of connective tissues and muscles. Enzymes improve the blood supply and the nutrient supply through the skin's dermal layer.

Healing Options

Home Remedies	• Neem • Sandalwood • Manjistha
Ayurvedic Supplements	• Neem Guard • Neem Guard body oil • Surakta • Raktasodhak Bati • Mahamanjishthadyarishta
Diet	• Drink an extra amount of water. • Bitter-tasting food should be taken regularly. • Avoid extra amounts of proteins and fat. • Avoid difficult-to-digest food. • Avoid food that irritates your skin.
Lifestyle	• Clean the body properly. • Exercise regularly. • Avoid excess sun exposure. • Avoid too many chemical-based creams. • Keep your space pollution-free.
Yoga	• Sarvangasan • Pranayam • Padahastasan • Halasan • Bhujangasan

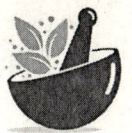

84

Sore Throat

Sore throat refers to the inflammation of the pharynx or the back of the throat. It occurs frequently when a person has a cold or an influenza attack. This inflammation may also involve the tonsils and adenoids.

Symptoms

In the case of an acute sore throat, the patient complains of pain, irritation and inflammation in the throat, followed by chills, fever and some hoarseness or laryngitis. The lymph glands along the side of the neck may become swollen and tender. The back of the throat may become red and even covered with a greyish-white membrane. The patient may experience difficulty swallowing, especially during the acute stage. There may be also some nasal discharge if the inflammation has spread to the nasal passage.

The main causes of a sore throat are common cold and influenza. Other causes include sinusitis, measles, diphtheria and even leukaemia in rare cases.

Healing Options

Home Remedies	• Mango bark • Cinnamon • Henna • Holy basil • Kantakari • Tamarind

| Ayurvedic Supplements | - Khadiradi Bati
- Lavangadi Bati
- Vyoshadi Bati |
|---|---|
| Diet | - A person suffering from a sore throat should fast on orange juice and water for three to five days, depending on the condition.
- When the severe symptoms subside, the patient may adopt an all-fruit diet for a further three or four days.
- Thereafter, adopt a well-balanced diet, with an emphasis on seeds, nuts, grains, raw vegetables and fresh fruits. |
| Lifestyle | - During the initial juice and water fast, the bowels should be cleansed daily with a warm water enema. This should be done twice daily in more serious cases.
- A wet pack should be applied to the throat at two-hourly intervals during the day and once at night.
- Gargling may be done several times a day. |
| Yoga | - Pranayam
- Surya Namaskar
- Meditation
- Ustrasan
- Singhasan
- Sasangasan |

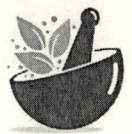

Sexual Impotence

Many people suffer from sexual dysfunction. The most common male sexual dysfunction is impotence.

Symptoms

Impotence takes three forms.

In primary impotence, the man's erectile dysfunction exists from the very beginning of sexual activity and he cannot have an erection.

Secondary impotence is the commonest and this implies that the man can normally attain an erection but fails on one or more occasions between normal activities.

The third form is associated with advancing age.

Root Causes

Sexual impotence may result from psychological illnesses such as depression, which lowers sex drive and erectile function. Tiredness, alcohol abuse, the therapeutic use of oestrogens, paralysis of the parasympathetic nerves by drugs or permanent damage to them and diabetes can also cause sexual impotence. Other causes of impotence include a devitalized condition of the system in general. The main problem of secondary impotence is the apprehension created by an earlier failure, which generates a good deal of anxiety.

Healing Options

| Home Remedies | - Garlic
- Onion
- Asparagus
- Drumstick
- Ginger
- Raisins |
|---|---|
| Ayurvedic Supplements | - Vigor 100 Stamina
- Vita-Ex (Gold)
- Musli Pak
- Chandraprabha Bati
- Shilajit capsules |
| Diet | - Adopt a fresh-fruit diet.
- Concentrate on food like nuts, cereals, vegetables, fruits, milk and honey.
- Avoid smoking, alcohol, tea, coffee and all processed, canned, refined and denatured food, especially white sugar and white flour and products made from them. |
| Lifestyle | - A vigorous massage of the body is highly beneficial in the treatment of impotence as it helps to revive muscular vigour, which is essential for nervous energy.
- The nerves of the genitals are controlled by the pelvic region. Hence, cold hip bath for ten minutes in the morning or evening is very effective. |
| Yoga | - Dhanurasan
- Sarvangasan
- Halasan
- Garurasan
- Sarvangasan |

Stomach Ulcer

A lesion between the stomach's inner lining and the duodenum is referred to as a stomach ulcer. A duodenal ulcer is located in the duodenum and a gastric ulcer in the stomach. Both are typically combined and referred to as stomach ulcers. According to Ayurveda, it is a tri-doshic ailment, meaning it affects the vata, pitta and kapha. However, pitta aggravation is observed in every instance.

Symptoms

Excruciating pain and discomfort in the upper abdomen are signs of a stomach ulcer. Pain from gastric ulcers usually occurs an hour after meals and rarely at night. When the stomach is empty between meals, duodenal ulcer discomfort typically manifests. Food, particularly milk, eases the pain. As the illness worsens, the stomach becomes distended as a result of excessive flatulence, emotional stress, sleeplessness and a slow deterioration of the body. Also, blood may be detected in the stool.

Root Causes

An increase in the stomach's hydrochloric acid leads to hyperacidity, which in turn causes a stomach ulcer. The stomach's inner lining is weakened by this potent acid, which is released by the cells of the stomach lining. The primary factors contributing to this disorder include smoking, drinking alcohol, coffee and eating large or spicy meals. Additional causes include gout, food poisoning, certain diseases, emotional disorders, stress and neurological tension, as well as the ingestion of certain medicines.

Ayurvedic Supplements	<ul><li>Acidity Guard</li><li>Diagest Guard Juice</li><li>Ayucid</li><li>Avipatikar Churna</li><li>Moti pisti</li></ul>
Diet	<ul><li>Since the main cause of stomach ulcers is hyperacidity, the first step is to avoid eating anything that makes the problem worse.</li><li>Spices, particularly chilli, and fried food ought to be avoided.</li><li>Milk should be freely taken, at intervals of three to four hours during a day, because the pain of the ulcer occurs at times when the stomach is empty. It is important to consume enough milk, wheat and ghee.</li></ul>
Lifestyle	<ul><li>In addition to the aforementioned, the patient must keep themselves free from the worries and stresses of life which are likely to exacerbate the ulcer pain.</li><li>Take sufficient rest and sleep for an hour every day.</li><li>It is important to make sure the patient can move the lower body because constipation can only make the problem worse.</li></ul>
Yoga	<ul><li>Gomukhasan</li><li>Vajrasan</li><li>Savasan</li></ul>

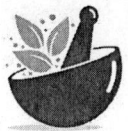

87

Skin Allergy

A skin allergy is the body's overreaction to one or more allergens. There are thousands of different allergens all around us and almost any substance can provoke an allergic reaction in someone (who is very sensitive) in our environment.

In Ayurveda the skin can be categorized into three types.

Vata skin is in general dry, thin and cool to the touch, easily gets dehydrated, and is very vulnerable to the influence of dry, windy weather.

Pitta skin is mostly fire, so this skin type tends to have more breakouts, photosensitivity, less tolerance to hot food and less tolerance to fiery temperament. Pitta skin looks ruddy and is warm to the touch. Pitta skin types tend to be more prone to freckles and moles than the other skin types.

Kapha skin is predominantly water and earth, so it tends to have all the qualities of water and earth; it can be greasy, thick and more tolerant to the sun.

Types of Skin Allergy

There are four main types of skin allergies, each caused by different allergens. Fortunately, there are many ways to relieve the symptoms. However, to choose an appropriate treatment, it's important to identify the type of allergy.

Contact dermatitis

The Greek word 'dermatitis' means 'inflammation of the skin' and is caused by touching a toxic substance. In most cases, the main symptom is a red rash, but it could be one of the several allergens that cause it, including metals, chemicals, rubber, plants and even pets.

Prickly heat

Warm weather often causes the itchy red rash known as prickly heat. The exact reason is not known, but it may be due to sweat getting trapped under the skin.

Bites and stings

Irritations from insect bites and stings can be uncomfortable, but reactions tend to be short-lived.

Urticaria

This type of allergy is often called nettle rash because it comes up as an itchy red rash, raised in the middle. Confusingly, it has nothing to do with stinging nettles at all, but is caused by eating a certain food or taking a particular drug.

Healing Options

Home Remedies	• Neem (*Azadiracta indica*) • Giloy (*Tinospora cordifolia*) • Manjistha (*Rubia cordifolia*) • Haridra (*Curcuma longa*)

Ayurvedic Supplements	• Allergy Guard • Immune Guard • Neem Guard • Surakta • Giloy Satwa
Diet	• Drink an extra amount of water. • Regularly eat bitter-tasting food. • Avoid extra amounts of proteins and fat. • Avoid difficult-to-digest food. • Avoid food that irritates your skin.
Lifestyle	• Clean the body regulary. • Exercise regularly. • Avoid excessive exposure to sun. • Avoid chemical-based creams. • Keep your room pollution-free.
Yoga	• Sarvangasan • Pranayam • Vajrasan • Ardha Kurmasan • Pawanmuktasan

Sciatica

Sciatica refers to pain in the back, which gradually spreads to the lower limbs. It is caused by the compression of the sciatic nerve near the lumbar region of the spine. This is known as *griddhasi* in Ayurveda. It occurs most frequently in people between 30 and 50 years of age.

Symptoms

- Pain and throbbing sensation in the rear of the leg
- Worsening pain during sitting or moving the affected limb
- Weakness, numbness, or difficulty in moving the leg or foot

Treatment (Non-Medicinal)

- Yoga
- Hip flexion and extension exercises
- Local hot fomentation
- Lumbosacral belts

Healing Options

Home Remedies	• Garlic (*Allium sativum*) • Guggulu (*Commiphora mukul*) • Giloy (*Tinospora cordifolia*) • Vatsanav (*Aconitum ferox*)

Ayurvedic Supplements	• Arth Plus • Arth Oil • Rumartho Gold • Rhuma Oil • Sinhanand Guggul • Kaishore Guggul
Diet	• Avoid curd and all sour food, pulses (except moong dal), rice, meat, fish, white bread, sugar, refined cereals, fried food, tea, or coffee. • Have potatoes and lemon juice. • Celery seeds and bitter gourd are highly beneficial.
Lifestyle	• Avoid lifting heavy weights. • Avoid sleeping on spongy mattresses. • Avoid squatting for too long. • Make dietary modifications, like adding high-fibre food, to ensure proper bowel evacuation. • Limit yourself to restricted exercise.
Yoga	• Halasan • Dhanurasan • Pawanmuktasan • Bhujangasan • Salavasan

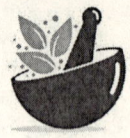

Syphilis

One of the most painful venereal diseases, syphilis is contagious and develops slowly and gradually.

Causes and Symptoms

Syphilis begins as a sore at the site of the infection and in its tertiary stage, shows changes which resemble the sores caused by leprosy and tuberculosis. In most cases, it is acquired via sexual intercourse with an infected person. The two main types of syphilis are acquired and inherited.

Acquired syphilis

It is caused by sexual intercourse with an infected person and sometimes by contact with the sores, or by using utensils or clothes of the patient.

This form of the disease has three stages—primary, secondary and tertiary. Sometimes these stages merge and the disease proceeds as a sequence of the various symptoms as the severity increases. Sometimes symptoms are so severe that ulcers appear all over the body.

Inherited syphilis

This disease may affect the child before its birth. It may even lead to a miscarriage or stillbirth. In some cases, the infant may start showing secondary symptoms after a few weeks of birth. They may develop deformity or deafness. If the symptoms are suppressed for a few years, the child may develop a sunken nose with a broad nasal bridge and may suffer from inflammation of the cornea or the iris.

Syphilis may manifest as painful boils on the prepuce of males or on the labia majora of the vagina among females. The eruptions turn into hard nodules and then subside, causing other symptoms.

Healing Options

Ayurvedic Supplements	• Ameer ras • Chopchinyadi churna
Diet and Lifestyle	The patients suffering from this disease should eat a salt-free diet.
Yoga	• Pawanmuktasan (Prevention purpose only) • Baddha Konasan (Prevention purpose only) • Viparit Karani (Prevention purpose only)

90
Sleeplessness

Sleep is essential for the normal, healthy functioning of the human body. Sleeplessness is usually associated with emotional or mental stress, anxiety, depression, work problems or financial stress. While sleeplessness is not usually related to any physical illness, there are some exceptions.

Any illness that causes pain or discomfort may cause sleeplessness. The more the mental stress, the more sleep is needed.

All the factors responsible for the aggravation of vayu and pitta in the human body can cause sleeplessness. Intake of spicy food and stimulating drinks, exercising immediately after meals, environmental factors like excessive heat, cold or rain, exposure to noise, and change of environment along with psychological factors lead to sleeplessness.

Effects of Lack of Sleep

- Simple tasks become difficult to accomplish
- Impaired short-term memory, concentration and alertness
- Increased chances of being in an accident
- Diminished ability to fight disease and repair tissue

You're probably not getting the sleep you need if you:

- feel groggy and lethargic in the morning,
- feel drowsy during the day,
- need more than 30 minutes to fall asleep, or
- wake up frequently at night and have trouble getting back to sleep.

Healing Options

| Ayurvedic Supplements | - Nightzz
- Stress Guard
- Brahmi capsules or tablets
- Sarpagandhaghan bati |
|---|---|
| **Diet and Lifestyle** | - Depending on the digestive capacity of the patients, they should be given a sufficiently nourishing diet. Heavy meals help with a good sleep.
- Buffalo milk, butter and ghee are considered very useful.
- Hot and spicy food should be avoided. |
| | **Tips for reducing sleeplessness**

- Plan more active days. A person who rests most of the day is likely to be awake at night. Discourage afternoon napping and plan activities such as walking.
- Monitor the diet. Restrict sweets and caffeine consumption to the morning hours. Have a light meal before bedtime.
- Seek medical advice if a physical ailment, such as bladder incontinence is making it difficult to sleep.
- Sometimes doctors prescribe medication to help the person relax at night.
- Change sleeping arrangements. Sleep in a different bedroom or wherever is more comfortable. Keep the room partially lit. |
| **Yoga** | - Gomukhasan
- Padahastasan
- Sarvangasan |

91
Stress

Stress can be defined as a state of worry or tension caused by a difficult situation. Stress is a natural human response that prompts us to address challenges and threats.

Stress is known as *sahasa* in Ayurveda. It causes *ojahksaya* (loss of immunity) and increases the susceptibility of the body to various diseases. Avoidance of stress is the best strategy for treatment, and where it is not possible, the body should be well-protected by taking appropriate care of one's diet and sleep, ensuring adequate rest as required by the body.

In terms of age, people from ages 18 to 34 have reported being most stressed about health and money, while adults from ages 35 to 64 reported increased chronic health and mental health issues as well as financial and economic stress.

Causes

Job-related stress: Excessive workload, deadlines, job insecurity and conflicts with colleagues or superiors are major causes for stress at a young age.

Financial stress: Debt, financial instability, or the inability to meet financial obligations can be a source of stress.

Relationship and family issues: Difficulties in personal relationships, conflicts with family members, marital problems, or caregiving responsibilities can lead to stress.

Major life changes: Significant life events such as moving to a new place, starting a new job, getting married, having a child, or experiencing the loss of a loved one can cause stress.

Health concerns: Dealing with chronic illnesses, acute health problems, or managing the health issues of loved ones can create stress.

Academic pressure: Students may experience stress due to academic expectations, exams, assignments, and the pressure to perform well.

Environmental factors: Stress can be triggered by factors like noise, pollution, overcrowding, or living in an unsafe neighbourhood.

Information overload: The constant exposure to a vast amount of information through technology and media can lead to stress and feelings of overwhelm.

Personal expectations: Setting unrealistic expectations for oneself, striving for perfection, or constantly seeking approval from others can create stress.

Traumatic events: Experiencing or witnessing a traumatic event such as an accident, natural disaster, or violence can lead to stress and post-traumatic stress disorder (PTSD).

Symptoms

- Fatigue and low energy levels
- Headaches and migraines
- Muscle tension and pain, including backaches and neck stiffness
- Digestive problems such as stomach aches, indigestion and irritable bowel syndrome (IBS)
- Anxiety, excessive worry and restlessness
- Irritability, mood swings and agitation
- Difficulty concentrating and making decisions
- Memory problems and forgetfulness

Healing Options

Home Remedies	- **Ashwagandha:** This herb, often referred to as the 'king of herbs', is renowned for its adaptogenic properties. Adaptogens are substances that help the body adapt to stress. - **Brahmi:** It is a known ayurvedic herb with medicinal properties used by practitioners for a long time. It can boost memory power and reduce anxiety. - **Tulsi:** It is one of the most common herbs that can be easily found in every Indian household. Also named holy basil, tulsi will give you a sense of calmness and has proven to be effective in the treatment of anxiety and stress. - **Jatamansi:** It is a known anti-stress ayurvedic medicine and helps in managing fatigue. According to Ayurvedic experts, the roots of jatamansi have therapeutic benefits. It keeps the mind and the body free from toxins and will give a sense of stability and a grounded feeling.
Ayurvedic Supplements	- Stress Guard - Stress Guard Anti-Stress Massage Oil - Ashwagandha tablets/capsules - Brahmi Bati
Diet	- Consume a wholesome and balanced diet that includes fresh, seasonal fruits, vegetables, whole grains and lean proteins. - Limit or avoid stimulants like caffeine and alcohol, as they can exacerbate stress and anxiety.

Lifestyle	• Regular physical activity such as walking, running, or playing sports can improve the mood, distract one from worries, and relieve tension and stress. • Exercise can also improve your general health. • Smoking or taking tobacco in any form should be given up completely.
Yoga	• Virasan • Vrikshasan • Trikonasan • Uttanasan • Uttana Shishosan • Matsyasan • Paschimottanasan

Tonsillitis (Inflammation of the Tonsils)

Tonsillitis is an acute inflammation of the tonsils, which are located on each side of the throat. Chronic tonsillitis is a term applied to cases where there is an enlargement of the tonsils accompanied by repeated infection.

Symptoms

The symptoms of tonsillitis are sore throat, fever, headache, pain in various parts of the body, difficulty swallowing and general weakness. The tonsils are visibly inflamed and red when the mouth is opened wide. Externally, the tonsillar lymph glands, which are just behind the angle of the jaw, are tender and enlarged. In severe cases, there is pain in the ear.

Root Causes

The chief cause of tonsillitis is a toxic condition of the system, which is brought to a head by a sudden lowering of vitality, resulting from sudden exposure to cold. The tonsils enlarge and get inflamed when the toxins are not removed through normal channels of elimination such as the bowels, kidneys and skin. A throat affliction of this kind is also associated with chronic constipation when the toxins are reabsorbed into the bloodstream.

Healing Options

Home Remedies	• Lime • Milk • Holy basil • Fenugreek seeds
Ayurvedic Supplements	• Dr Honey • Kasamrit Herbal • Khadiradi Bati • Lakshmivilas Ras
Diet	• To begin with, follow a liquid diet that includes fruit and vegetable juices, milk and soups. • After the acute symptoms subside, the patient should adopt a well-balanced diet containing grains, fats, proteins, vegetables and fruits.
Lifestyle	• Daily dry friction and hip bath as well as breathing and other exercises should form part of the health regimen. • The bowels should be cleansed daily. • Gargle with hot water and salt thrice a day.
Yoga	• Pranayam • Meditation • Ustrasan • Sasangasan • Singhasan

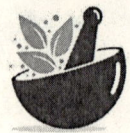

Toothache

Toothache usually refers to pain around the teeth or jaw. In most instances, toothaches are caused by tooth or jaw problems, such as a dental cavity, a cracked tooth, an exposed tooth root, gum disease, disease of the jaw joint (temporomandibular joint), or a spasm of the muscles used for chewing. The severity of a toothache can range from chronic and mild to sharp and excruciating. The pain may be aggravated by chewing or by cold or heat.

Causes of Toothache

The common dental causes of toothache include dental cavities, dental abscess, gum disease, irritation of the tooth root, cracked tooth syndrome, temporomandibular disease, impaction and eruption.

Dental cavities

Dental cavities (caries) are holes in the two outer layers of a tooth called enamel and dentin. The enamel is the outermost white, hard surface and the dentin is the yellow layer just beneath the enamel. Both layers protect the inner tooth tissue called pulp, which contains blood vessels and nerves. Certain bacteria in the mouth convert simple sugars into acid. The acid softens and (along with saliva) dissolves the enamel and dentin, creating cavities.

Gum disease

Gum disease refers to the inflammation of the soft tissue (gingiva) and an abnormal loss of the bone that surrounds the teeth and holds them in place. Gum disease is caused by toxins secreted by bacteria in plaque, which accumulate over time along the gumline. This plaque is a mixture of food, saliva and bacteria. An early symptom of gum disease is bleeding gums without pain.

A toothache can be caused by a problem that does not originate from a tooth or the jaw.

Healing Options

Herbal Home Remedies	• Clove • Holy basil • Babul
Ayurvedic Supplements	• Dant Manjan Lal • Clove oil • Irimedadi Taila • Lavangadi Bati
Yoga	• Singhasan • Ardha Chandrasan • Vajrasan

94

Underweight
(Less than Normal Weight)

Being thin, underweight or overweight is a relative term based on the ideal weight for a given height, built and sex. A person is considered moderately underweight if he or she weighs 10 per cent below the ideal body weight, and markedly so if the weight is 20 per cent below the ideal body weight.

TABLE 1
IDEAL HEIGHT AND WEIGHT FOR MEN

Height Feet Inches	Small Frame	Medium Frame	Large Frame
5'2"	128–134	131–141	138–150
5'3"	130–136	133–143	140–153
5'4"	132–138	135–145	142–156
5'5"	134–140	137–148	144–160
5'6"	136–142	139–151	146–164
5'7"	138–145	142–154	149–168
5'8"	140–148	145–157	152–172
5'9"	142–151	148–160	155–176
5'10"	144–154	151–163	158–180
5'11"	146–157	154–166	161–184
6'0"	149–160	157–170	164–188
6'1"	152–164	160–174	168–192

6'2"	155–168	164–178	172–197
6'3"	158–172	167–182	176–202
6'4"	162–176	171–187	181–207

*Weights at ages 25–59 based on lowest mortality. Weight in pounds according to frame (in indoor clothing weighing 5 lbs, shoes with 1 inch heels).

TABLE 2
IDEAL HEIGHT AND WEIGHT FOR WOMEN

Height Feet Inches	Small Frame	Medium Frame	Large Frame
4'10"	102–111	109–121	118–131
4'11"	103–113	111–123	120–134
5'0"	104–115	113–126	122–137
5'1"	106–118	115–129	125–140
5'2"	108–121	118–132	128–143
5'3"	111–124	121–135	131–147
5'4"	114–127	124–138	134–151
5'5"	117–130	127–141	137–155
5'6"	120–133	130–144	140–159
5'7"	123–136	133–147	143–163
5'8"	126–139	136–150	146–167
5'9"	129–142	139–153	149–170
5'10"	132–145	142–156	152–173
5'11"	135–148	145–159	155–176
6'0"	138–151	148–162	158–179

*Weights at ages 25–59 based on lowest mortality. Weight in pounds according to frame (in indoor clothing weighing 5 lbs, shoes with 1 inch heels).

Symptoms

Thinness due to an inadequate calorie intake is a serious condition, especially in young people. They often feel easily fatigued, have poor physical stamina and low resistance to infections. Diseases like tuberculosis, respiratory disorders, pneumonia, heart diseases, cerebral haemorrhage, nephritis, typhoid fever and cancer are quite common among them.

Causes

Thinness may be due to inadequate nutrition or excessive bodily activity, or both. Emotional factors or bad eating habits such as skipping meals, small meals, habitual fasting and inadequate exercise can also be among the reasons. Other factors include inadequate digestion and absorption of food due to wrong dietary patterns for a particular metabolism, metabolic disturbances such as overactive thyroid, and hereditary tendencies. Disorders such as chronic dyspepsia, chronic diarrhoea, intestinal worms, liver disorders, diabetes mellitus, insomnia, constipation and sexual disorders can also lead to thinness.

Healing Options

Home Remedies	• Muskmelon • Mango milk • Milk • Figs • Raisins • High-nutrient diet
Ayurvedic Supplements	• Zest Men • Zest Women • Spirulina Plus • Musli capsules

Diet	- Underweight people should eat frequent small meals, as they tend to feel full quickly.
- To gain weight, the diet should include more calories than used in daily activities to allow accumulation of body fat. The allowance of 500 calories above the daily average needs is enough for a weight gain of ½ kg weekly.
- All refined food containing white flour and sugar should be avoided.
Lifestyle	Regular exercises such as walking, dancing, yoga, meditation and massage are important as they serve as relaxants, reduce stress and induce good sleep.
Yoga	- Sarvangasan
- Halasan
- Matsyasan
- Padahastasan
- Vajrasan
- Pawanmuktasan

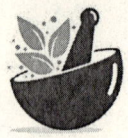

Urinary Tract Diseases

The urinary tract comprises the kidneys, ureters, bladder and urethra. These organs work together to produce, transport, store and excrete urine.

Urine contains the by-products of the body's metabolism, salts, toxins and water. For instance, blood, protein, or white blood cells in the urine may indicate an injury, infection or inflammation of the kidneys. Glucose in the urine may be an indication of diabetes.

Problems in the urinary system can be caused by ageing, illness or injury. As you get older, changes in the structure of the kidneys cause them to lose some of their ability to remove wastes from the blood. Also, the muscles in the ureters, bladder and urethra tend to lose some of their strength. Some people may have more urinary infections because the bladder muscles do not tighten enough to empty the bladder completely. A decrease in the strength of muscles of the sphincters and the pelvis can also cause incontinence, the unwanted leakage of urine. Illness or injury can also prevent the kidneys from filtering the blood completely or block the passage of urine.

Burning

While passing urine, some people feel a burning sensation in the urinary passage. It may be due to an infection in the urinary tract like gonorrhoea, enlargement of the prostate, a stone in the urinary bladder, or the urine being concentrated. The burning sensation may occur during the passage of urine or after that. It may subside by taking alkaline drinks or water.

Haematuria

The presence of blood in the urine is called haematuria. According to Ayurveda, it is a form of *adhoga rakta pitta*. It is commonly caused by stones or infections in the genital-urinary tract and some haemorrhagic conditions.

Nephritis

This refers to inflammation of the kidney. It is of several types and the different stages of the disease produce distinct symptoms. In Ayurveda it is called *vrikka shotha*. Usually, there is oedema of the face, which is more prominent in the morning and slowly subsides as the day passes on. The person's blood pressure may increase and they may suffer from biliousness, nausea, vomiting, abdominal pain, headache and diarrhoea.

Bedwetting

It is the involuntary urination at night. Children after the age of three or four years normally possess sufficient control over their urinary sphincters. Because of certain reasons, this control does not manifest and they continue to wet their bed at night. This continues in some cases even up to the age of 15. Both boys and girls can suffer from this ailment.

Kidney stones

Urinary stones are generally formed by calcium, phosphates or oxalates. The stones are formed primarily in the kidneys and sometimes go unnoticed for a long time. In certain circumstances, they slowly dissolve or become lodged in a narrow part of the tract, causing excruciating pain.

Stones are formed in the body because of vayu. It creates dryness in the body which causes the chemicals to accumulate over the nucleus, which ultimately takes the shape of a stone. At times the entire kidney is filled with these stones and calcifies and stops functioning. If urine is not excreted through the kidneys, or excreted in small quantities, uraemia sets in and causes many complications. The same phenomenon takes place if a piece of stone gets lodged in the ureter or bladder. The patient may experience pain in the lumbar region.

Urinary tract infections

Certain bacteria cause infection of the urinary tract. Women are more susceptible to UTIs than men. Drinking fluids can help flush out the bacteria. An infection in the urinary bladder is called cystitis. If the infection is in one or both kidneys, it is called pyelonephritis.

Prostatitis

It is an inflammation of the prostate gland that causes frequent urination, burning or painful urination (dysuria), and pain in the lower back and genital area. In some cases, prostatitis is caused by a bacterial infection. The more common forms of prostatitis are not associated with any known infecting organism.

Proteinuria

It is the presence of abnormal amounts of protein in the urine. Healthy kidneys take waste out of the blood but leave the protein. Protein in the urine does not cause a problem in itself, but it may be a sign that the kidneys are not working properly.

Healing Options

Herbal Remedies	• Shilajit (*Mineral Pitch, Asphaltum*) • Gokshura (*Tribulus terrestris*) • Punarnava (*Boerrhavia diffusa*) • Guduchi (*Tinospora cordifolia*) • Chandan (*Santalum album*)
Ayurvedic Supplements	• Chandraprabha Bati • Gokshuradi Guggulu • Shilajit tablets ot capsules • Chandanasava
Diet	• Hot spices are to be strictly avoided. • The patient should be given as much water as possible to drink. • Fresh lemon juice, fresh coconut water, orange juice, sugarcane juice and pineapple juice are extremely useful in this condition. • The patient should be given fruits like apples, grapes, peaches and plums in good quantity.
Lifestyle	• The patient should not expose himself to the sun or heat. Excessive perspiration removes a lot of water from the body and the urine becomes concentrated. Passage of this concentrated urine through the urinary tract causes irritation and a burning sensation.
Yoga	• Gomukhasan • Pawanmuktasan • Ardha Matsendrasan • Ardha Chandrasan • Janushirasan • Supta Bhadrasan

Urticaria

This is a vascular reaction of the skin characterized by the transient appearance of elevated patches that are redder or paler than the surrounding skin and often accompanied by itching. In Ayurveda this is called *shita pitta*.

The causes of this disease are allergens or taking a cold bath immediately after exercise when the body is hot. Intestinal worms and exposure to the cold wind often cause urticaria. The patches appear all over the body suddenly or gradually. There may be severe itching. The patient may get attacks of cold, cough, bronchitis and stomach disorder.

Treatments

Haridra is one of the most popular household remedies for urticaria. It is given to the patient in the form of a paste by triturating its powder with water in a dose of two teaspoonfuls three times a day. It has a slightly bitter taste. So, it could be given by mixing it with milk and sugar. A palatable preparation of Haridra is known as Haridra Khanda. It is available in the form of granules and can be given to the patient in a dose of two teaspoonfuls three times a day followed by a cup of warm water.

Gairika (red ochre) is also popularly used in this condition. After processing, it is given in a dose of one teaspoonful three times a day mixed with honey. Kamadugha Rasa, which contains gairika in a significantly large quantity, is also given to the patient in a dose of 0.5 g four times a day with honey.

During an acute attack of this disease, Suta, Shekhara Rasa and Arogya Vardhini Rasa can be given to the patient. Both these medicines either individually or in compound form are given in a dose of 0.5 g three times a day mixed with honey.

If the patient is constipated, he may be given the powder of haritaki in a dose of two teaspoonfuls at bedtime with hot water.

Healing Options

Herbal Home Remedy	• Neem • Harida • Drumstick • Haritaki
Ayurvedic Supplements	• Neem Guard • Immune Guard • Allergy Guard • Neem oil • Haridra Khanda
Diet	• The patient should be given a salt-free diet as far as possible. Sour food like curd is prohibited. Bitter vegetables like bitter gourd and bitter variety of drumstick are useful in this condition. Onion and garlic can be given to the patient in good quantity.
Lifestyle	• During acute attacks of urticaria, the patient should be massaged with mustard oil mixed with the powder of rock salt. Thereafter, the whole body should be exposed to the sun and gently rubbed with a copper coin. This gives instant relief. If there are worms in the intestine then it should be treated. Otherwise, urticaria will recur.

Yoga	• Sarvangasan
	• Halasan
	• Padahastasan
	• Pavanmuktasan
	• Bhujangasan

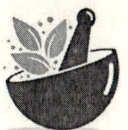

Vertigo

In Ayurveda vertigo is referred to as *brahma*, where vitiated pitta combines with vitiated vata to cause a spinning sensation.

Vertigo, or dizziness, refers to the sensation of spinning or whirling that occurs as a result of disturbance in balance. It may also be described as a feeling of dizziness or lightheadedness.

Causes

The most common causes of vertigo are illnesses that affect the inner ear. Vertigo can manifest in various forms.

Benign positional vertigo: In this condition a change in the position of the head causes a sudden spinning sensation.

Acute labyrinthitis: This is due to the imbalance of the inner ear.

Meniere's disease: It is a condition where a change in volume of fluid in the inner ear causes vertigo.

Symptoms

- Spinning sensation or imbalance
- Lightheadedness
- Nausea
- Vomiting
- Tinnitus (ringing of the ear)

Healing Options

Home Remedies	• Giloy (*Tinospora cordifolia*) • Pitpapda (*Fumaria officinalis*) • Vacha (*Acorus calamus*) • Yavasa (*Alhagi pseudalhagi*) • Sariva (*Hemidesmus indicus*)
Ayurvedic Supplements	• Zest Men • Zest Women • Sarivadi Bati • Prawalpisti • Giloy Satwa
Diet	• Eat plenty of green vegetables. • Eat seasonal fruits. • Avoid extra amount of salt. • Avoid junk food as much as possible.
Lifestyle	• Practise breathing relaxation. • Avoid tobacco and alcohol. • Try to sleep without pillow.
Yoga	• Halasan (Plough pose) • Dhanurasan (Bow pose) • Tadasan (for prevention purpose) • Vrikshasan (for prevention purpose) • Ardha Koti Chakrasan (for prevention purpose)

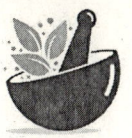

Women and Obesity

Weight gain or obesity in women can be caused by several natural or environmental factors.

Some women gain weight due to biological changes during and after pregnancy. Misconceptions about the needs of a pregnant woman, such as eating double the amount of food to bear and feed her child, are sometimes responsible for such changes.

Some women tend to gain weight during menopause. Due to hormonal imbalance, obesity sets in, even though they had maintained normal weight previously.

Obesity is also caused when the pituitary gland secretion is deficient. In cases where this gland is overactive and secretes more hormones than it should, the person grows to an abnormal size. This is known as gigantism. The second gland that contributes to obesity is the thyroid, which is located in the neck.

The adrenal glands are located above the kidneys. The hormones secreted by these glands control our emotions like anger, fear, etc. Excessive secretion of these hormones, or when these hormones are administered in massive doses, cause a severe disorder known as Cushing's Syndrome or the Moon Face syndrome.

The affected person bloats to abnormal proportions and becomes a victim of various other disorders like hypertension and diabetes.

The pancreas is a very important digestive organ that secretes the pancreatic juice and an essential endocrine hormone, insulin. Insulin is essential in sugar metabolism. The fat stored from refined carbohydrates and sugar due to the abnormal sugar metabolism results in obesity.

In some cases, if the sex hormones secreted by the ovaries in females are deficient during menopause, it results in obesity. Administering hormones further adds to the bulk. This is the case after hysterectomy in some women.

Overeating is another serious problem that causes obesity.

Causes

- Dietary and lifestyle changes
- Weight gain after childbirth
- Use of oral contraceptives
- Menopause
- Stress
- Binge eating
- Hormonal imbalance
- Endocrine disorders

Healing Options

Herbal Home Remedies	• Ginger tea • Cumin water • Cinnamon • Fennel seeds
Ayurvedic Supplements	• Ezislim Juice • Ezislim capsules • Isabgol • Shilajit • Triphala Juice

Diet	• Eat fruits, vegetables and salads.
	• Always consume a little less than you are hungry for.
	• Avoid dinner after 8 p.m.
	• Avoid over-processed food.
	• Avoid excess sugar and salt.
Lifestyle	• Stay physically active.
	• Exercise regularly.
	• Eat healthy food.
	• Manage stress.
Yoga	• Surya Namaskar
	• Pawanmuktasan
	• Gomukasan

Warts (Superficial Growths on the Skin)

Warts refer to hard growths on the skin. They are common in both children and adults. Warts spread rather quickly, but are usually harmless. They also disappear spontaneously.

Symptoms

Warts have various shapes and sizes and usually appear as rough bumps on the skin. These bumps appear more frequently on the fingers, elbows, knees, face and scalp. Those that appear on the soles of the feet are called plantar warts. They are very painful, leaving the person unable to walk properly.

Causes

The main cause of warts is a viral infection of the skin. Plantar warts on the soles are usually contracted in swimming pools. Constitutional factors, however, appear to be at the root of the trouble. These factors lead to some defects in the proper development of the skin surface in certain areas.

Healing Options

Herbal Home Remedies	• Castor oil • Potato • Onion • Marigold • Cashew nut oil
Ayurvedic Supplements	• Neem Guard • Surakta • Raktasodhak Bati • Sarivadyarishta
Diet	• The patient should take fruit juice, fresh fruits and vegetables. Papayas, pears, oranges and mangoes are recommended.
Lifestyle	• Clean your skin properly. • Exercise and sweat it out. • Wear clean clothes daily.
Yoga	• Light free-hand exercise • Sarvangasan • Halasan • Sasangasan

Whooping Cough

This is known as *dushta kasa* in Ayurveda. It is an infectious bacterial disease that occurs mainly in children.

Causes and Symptoms

In the beginning, whooping cough is marked by catarrh of the nose, sneezing, watery eyes, irritation of the throat, feverishness and cough. Later, the symptoms of catarrh disappear, but the cough becomes more persistent. The cough is marked by paroxysms of coughing, consisting of a series of violent and rapid expiratory coughs, succeeded by a loud, sonorous or crowing inspiration—the whoop. Hence the name, whooping cough. The child's face can sometimes turn blue because the paroxysm deprives the lungs of air. Children are usually more susceptible to this malady than adults. According to Ayurveda, whooping cough is the result of a disturbance of the vata dosha in the body.

Healing Options

Ayurvedic Supplements	<ul><li>Dr. Honey</li><li>Kasamrit Herbal</li><li>Sitopaladi churna</li><li>Kantakaryaveleh</li><li>Vasavleha</li></ul>

Home Remedies	Juice of ginger, with an equal quantity of honey, should be taken twice a day.
Diet and Lifestyle	• The patient must be protected against exposure and sudden colds as they are liable to aggravate his condition and hamper quick recovery.
Yoga	• Ardha Kurmasan • Bhujangasan • Dhanurasan